Innovations in Nursing Education:
Building the Future of Nursing

Edited by:
Linda Caputi, EdD, RN, CNE, ANEF

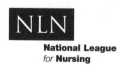

National League
for **Nursing**

Wolters Kluwer | Lippincott Williams & Wilkins
Health
Philadelphia · Baltimore · New York · London
Buenos Aires · Hong Kong · Sydney · Tokyo

Acquisitions Editor: Christina Burns
Product Development Editor: Eve Malakoff-Klein
Production Project Manager: Joan Sinclair
Designer: Stephen Druding
Illustration: Jennifer Clements
Manufacturing Coordinator: Karin Duffield
Composition: Aptara, Inc.
Printer: DRC

351 West Camden Street   Two Commerce Square/2001 Market Street
Baltimore, MD 21201   Philadelphia, PA 19103

9 8 7 6 5 4 3 2 1

Printed in the United States

Library of Congress Cataloging-in-Publication Data

Innovations in nursing education : building the future of nursing /
Linda Caputi, editor ; illustrations by Jennifer Clements.
    p. ; cm.
Includes bibliographical references.
ISBN 978-1-934758-18-2 (alk. paper)
  I. Caputi, Linda, editor of compilation.   II. National League for
Nursing, issuing body.
  [DNLM: 1. Education, Nursing–organization & administration.
2. Education, Nursing–trends. WY 18]
  RT76
  610.73071′1–dc23
                                    2013031359

Disclaimer
Care has been taken to confirm the accuracy of the information presented and to describe generally accepted practices. However, the authors, editors, and publisher are not responsible for errors or omissions or for any consequences from application of the information in this book and make no warranty, expressed or implied, with respect to the currency, completeness, or accuracy of the contents of the publication. Application of this information in a particular situation remains the professional responsibility of the practitioner; the clinical treatments described and recommended may not be considered absolute and universal recommendations.

The authors, editors, and publisher have exerted every effort to ensure that drug selection and dosage set forth in this text are in accordance with the current recommendations and practice at the time of publication. However, in view of ongoing research, changes in government regulations, and the constant flow of information relating to drug therapy and drug reactions, the reader is urged to check the package insert for each drug for any change in indications and dosage and for added warnings and precautions. This is particularly important when the recommended agent is a new or infrequently employed drug.

Some drugs and medical devices presented in this publication have Food and Drug Administration (FDA) clearance for limited use in restricted research settings. It is the responsibility of the health care provider to ascertain the FDA status of each drug or device planned for use in his or her clinical practice.

To purchase additional copies of this book, call our customer service department at (800) 638-3030 or fax orders to (301) 223-2320. International customers should call (301) 223-2300. Visit Wolters Kluwer Health | Lippincott Williams & Wilkins online at www.lww.com. Visit the National League for Nursing online at www.nln.org.

Contributors

ABOUT THE EDITOR

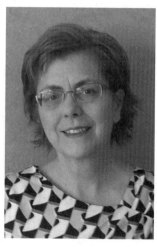

Dr. Linda Caputi, EdD, RN, CNE, ANEF, is the editor of the *Innovation Center,* a column in the National League for Nursing's journal *Nursing Education Perspectives*. She is a Certified Nurse Educator, and a fellow in the NLN's Academy of Nursing Education. Dr. Caputi is Professor Emerita, College of DuPage, and most recently taught in an online Master's in Nursing Education program. She has won six awards for teaching excellence from Sigma Theta Tau and is included in three different years in the *Who's Who Among America's Teachers*. The second edition of her book *Teaching Nursing: The Art and Science* was selected as the winner of the 2010 Top Teaching Tools Award in the print category from the *Journal of Nursing Education*. She has recently completed a three-year term on the NLN's Board of Governors.

Dr. Caputi is also president of Linda Caputi, Inc., a nursing education consulting company, and has worked with hundreds of nursing programs over the last 20 years on topics related to revising curriculum, transforming clinical education, test-item writing and test construction, using an evidence-based model for NCLEX® success, assisting with accreditation, and numerous other nursing education topics.

ABOUT THE CONTRIBUTORS

Deborah S. Adelman, PhD, RN, NE-BC, is a professor of nursing at Kaplan University in the MSN program. She has worked in nursing education for over 25 years and has taught online since 1994. She has designed nursing courses and programs online from the ADN to the doctoral level. In her role as interim MSN academic chair, Deborah created writing groups that produced published articles and research studies at Kaplan among online BSN and MSN faculty.

Katherine B. Ardoin, MSN, RN, CNE, is an instructor at the University of Louisiana at Lafayette College of Nursing and Allied Health Professions. For 18 years, Katherine worked as a staff nurse on various medical-surgical units and then as a nursing staff development specialist. For the past 5 years, Katherine has provided clinical teaching to first-semester junior nursing students on medical-surgical units and classroom instruction to sophomores, teaching therapeutic communication.

Carrie A. Bailey, MSN, RN, ACNS-BC, has a master's degree in nursing and is a PhD candidate in educational psychology and research, adult learning at The University of

Tennessee in Knoxville, TN. She has practiced nursing for 14 years and is an adult health clinical nurse specialist. Throughout her nursing career, Carrie has continued to teach both graduate and undergraduate nursing students in the clinical setting.

Lance Baily, BA, EMT, has been called a "thought leader" in the industry of medical simulation. With a background in audiovisual production, computers, and Emergency Medical Services/Fire Service, Lance has previously served as a simulation technician to the LA Harbor College District and as founding director of the Clinical Simulation Center of Las Vegas. Today, as an entrepreneur, Lance continues the work he pioneered with HealthySimulation.com, SimGHOSTS.org, and HealthySimAdmin.com.

Miriam E. Bar-on, MD, FAAP, is the associate dean for graduate medical education and professor of pediatrics at the University of Nevada School of Medicine in Las Vegas, NV. She serves as one of three deans in the administration of the Clinical Simulation Center of Las Vegas. Miriam has been a medical educator for over 25 years and is involved professionally in multiple national organizations in leadership roles. She has done multiple presentations regionally, nationally, and internationally, both research and medical education oriented.

Amy M. Barrett, MSN, MEd, RN, works on the Care Gaps, Patient Education and Outreach Program at Geisinger Medical Center in Danville, PA. Prior to coming to Geisinger, Amy served as a full-time faculty member in the practical nursing program at Clearfield County Career and Technology Center, Clearfield, PA, and as temporary adjunct faculty at Clarion University, Venango campus, Oil City, PA. Amy was the education director at the former Philipsburg Area Hospital, expanding staff development programs and career ladder, and overseeing all hospital-based education programs.

Kelly M. Bower, PhD, RN, APHN-BC, is an instructor at Johns Hopkins University School of Nursing in Baltimore, MD. She is a public health nurse with years of practice experience at community agencies and clinics serving vulnerable populations in Baltimore City. Kelly's years of clinical practice have contributed to her expertise in conducting community health needs assessments, authoring successful grant applications, and designing and implementing program evaluation. Kelly's area of scholarly work is focused on neighborhood physical and social determinants of health and the impact on racial health inequities in urban populations.

Sarah Brittain Dysart, MA, is coordinator of learning technologies in the Faculty Center for Ignatian Pedagogy at Loyola University Chicago. She works closely with faculty and staff to explore, apply, and evaluate technological solutions that enhance students' academic experience. Sarah co-developed and helps teach Loyola's online teaching course, an intensive course that prepares faculty for all aspects of transitioning a course from the face-to-face to online environment. She specializes in providing assistance to Science, Technology, Engineering, and Mathematics (STEM) instructors, and as such, shares the university's strategy for preparing online STEM instructors through various conference presentations, the Sloan Consortium's effective practices online repository, and through consultations with instructors and administrators at other domestic and international institutions.

Vicki J. Brownrigg, PhD, RN, FNP-C, is an assistant professor in the Clinical Teaching Track and is doctorate of nursing practice program coordinator at Beth-El College of Nursing and Health Sciences at the University of Colorado, Colorado Springs. In addition to her 20 years of teaching, she has 30 years of practice in acute and primary care settings. This combination of being both a nurse educator and a practicing nurse has resulted in a strong commitment to ensure that nursing education programs reflect current trends in health care. As an NLN Health Information Technology scholar, Vicki is committed to preparing nursing graduates with the requisite knowledge and skills to embrace and wisely employ new and promising health care technologies.

Toni Bromley, MS, RN, is a nursing instructor at Rogue Community College, Grants Pass, OR. Toni has 17 years of teaching nursing in associate degree programs. She has been active with the Oregon Consortium for Nursing Education (OCNE) since its inception and is currently the co-chair of the OCNE Learning Activities Committee.

Lisa M. Ciampini, MS, served as graduate assistant at Austin Peay State University School of Nursing in Clarksville, TN, from fall 2010 to fall 2011. During this time she assisted the director of the school of nursing on several projects including research and editing on "A BSN Action Guide for Responding to 2011 Institute of Medicine Recommendations." Lisa has a bachelor's degree from Marymount University and graduated in spring 2012 from Austin Peay State University with a master's degree in school counseling.

Mary Jane Cook, MSN, RN, FNP, BC, is a PhD student at Indiana University and a faculty member at the College of Nursing at Michigan State University, East Lansing, MI. She teaches in the nurse practitioner and doctorate of nursing practice programs. Her research interest is graduate nursing education and instructional systems technology. She has participated in the design and piloting of a virtual pediatric clinic on Spartan Health Island in Second Life. Mary Jane also practices as a family nurse practitioner at the MSU Family Health Center.

Elizabeth Ellen Cooper, DNP, RN, CNE, CNL, is an assistant professor in the School of Nursing and Health Professions at the University of San Francisco. In addition to teaching and advising undergraduate nursing students, Elizabeth created the position of quality and safety officer. By providing a transparent look to safety in the school, bringing safety threads into all clinical courses, and including health care institutions into the discussion, Elizabeth hopes to help students graduate with a clear picture of safety issues, the importance of transparency, and the feeling of the presence of a just culture in health care with the safety of our patients as the most important point.

Deborah P. Copeland, PhD, RN, is a full-time nursing professor at Palm Beach State College, Lake Worth, FL. Her present emphasis is medical-surgical nursing and clinical simulation; however, she possesses over 38 years of varied experience in medical-surgical nursing, oncology, nursing supervision, quality management, and nursing education. Deborah's most recent efforts focus on the development, implementation, and evaluation of intentional learning experiences designed to enhance nursing students' competencies to care for the older adult population in various clinical settings.

C. Amelia Davis, PhD, is an assistant professor of educational research at Georgia Southern University, Statesboro, GA. Her area of interest includes qualitative research, particularly arts-based research and performance ethnography, in adult education settings. At the time this research was completed, Amelia was a PhD candidate in educational psychology and research, adult learning, at The University of Tennessee.

Katherine J. Dontje, PhD, RN, FNP, is a faculty member at the College of Nursing at Michigan State University, East Lansing, MI. She earned her BSN and master's degree from Michigan State University and her PhD from University of Wisconsin Milwaukee with a focus on patient self-management and informatics. She is director of graduate clinical programs at the college and teaches in the nurse practitioner and doctorate of nursing practice programs. Her research interests have focused on working with both providers and patients to make shared decisions about treatment options for chronic conditions.

Mary Enzman-Hines, PhD, APRN, CNS, CPNP, APHN-BC, is professor emerita at the Beth El College of Nursing and Health Sciences at the University of Colorado, Colorado Springs (UCCS) and a certified pediatric nurse practitioner at WEE Care Pediatrics in Colorado Springs, CO. For over 30 years, Mary was a professor of nursing in the UCCS graduate program and most recently was the DNP program coordinator. Mary was lead faculty in the development of the holistic conceptual framework for the entire nursing program. Additionally, Mary co-created the family nurse practitioner and the holistic clinical nurse specialist tracts within the graduate program and the DNP framed with caring philosophy and reflection. Mary received Health Resources and Services Administration (HRSA) grant funding for the implementation of the DNP. Mary is the immediate past president for the American Holistic Nurses Association and a HIT scholar through NLN.

David Frommer, AIA, NCARB, is executive director of planning and construction at the University of Nevada, Las Vegas (UNLV). David also has served or is serving in the following roles: as an adjunct instructor of architecture at the UNLV School of Architecture, as president of the American Institute of Architects (AIA) Nevada and Las Vegas chapters, as the chair of the AIA National Public Architects Knowledge Committee, as a member of the Editorial Board of Architecture Las Vegas magazine, as co-chair of the 2013 Design-Build Institute of America National Conference Planning Committee, and on a variety of design/construction and service award juries.

Priscilla K. Gazarian, PhD, RN, is an assistant professor at Simmons College, School of Nursing and Health Sciences, and a nursing program director and nurse scientist in the Center for Nursing Excellence at Brigham and Women's Hospital. With over 20 years of experience as a nurse educator, she has presented and published on innovative teaching strategies. Priscilla is an expert in the use cognitive task analysis methods to describe nurses' clinical decision-making and has received funding for the development of simulation scenarios directed at aiding nurses in the early recognition of changes in patient condition. These projects resulted in the development of two simulation scenarios related to the early recognition and treatment of delirium and stroke among hospitalized patients.

Kathryn L. Gramling, PhD, RN, is newly retired from an associate professorship at University of Massachusetts Dartmouth. Kathy began teaching in Madison, WI, in the late 1960s. Kathy's doctoral study was completed at the University of Colorado. Her research interest is in the art of nursing and her teaching passion is promoting theory-guided practice.

Gail Hanson, MSN, RN, is an instructor in the Niehoff School of Nursing at Loyola University Chicago. Gail has been an educator since 1991, teaching undergraduate and graduate nursing students. In her role at Loyola, she teaches undergraduate nursing students theory in the classroom and application of the nursing process in the clinical setting. She has a current research interest in quality and safety initiatives, and has presented nationally on the application of the Quality and Safety Education for Nurses (QSEN) process within the inpatient psychiatric setting.

Pamela R. Jeffries, PhD, RN, FAAN, ANEF, professor and associate dean for academic affairs at Johns Hopkins University School of Nursing in Baltimore, MD, is nationally known for her research and work in developing simulations and online teaching and learning. Pamela is well regarded for her expertise in experiential learning, innovative teaching strategies, new pedagogies, and the delivery of content using technology in nursing education. She is a fellow of the American Academy of Nursing (FAAN), an American Nurse Educator fellow (ANEF), a Robert Wood Johnson Foundation executive nurse fellow (ENF), a member of the Institute of Medicine's global intraprofessional education (IPE) forum, and has just been appointed as president-elect to the interprofessional, international Society for Simulation in Healthcare (SSH).

Sharon J. Kinney, MSN, RN, CNE, is a full-time faculty member in the associate degree nursing program at Central Maine Community College, Auburn, ME. Previously, Sharon was a nursing instructor in the practical nursing program at the Clearfield County Career and Technology Center and in the associate degree nursing program at Lock Haven University of Pennsylvania. She has been teaching nursing since 1993 and became an NLN certified nurse educator in 2008.

Cheryl B. Krieg, MSN, RNC-OB, is the simulation coordinator at the Clearfield County Career and Technology Center (CCCTC) practical nursing program, Clearfield, PA. Cheryl has been using simulation to enhance the learning of the CCCTC practical nursing students since 2007. Cheryl has worked as an RN staff nurse since 1991 and as an obstetrical nurse since 1994.

Timothy J. Legg, PhD, RN-BC, CRNP, GNP-BC, CNE, is professor and interim academic chair of the master of science in nursing program at Kaplan University, Chicago, IL. He maintains clinical practice as a nurse practitioner specializing in geropsychiatric care. Additionally, he is the secretary for the Pennsylvania chapter of the American Psychiatric Nurses Association as well as a member of the continuing education reviewer unit for the Pennsylvania State Nurses Association.

Elsie Maurer, MSN, RN, NEA-BC, is the nursing program director at the Clearfield County Career and Technology Center's practical nursing program in Clearfield, PA. Elsie has been involved in nursing education at the practical nurse and associate degree levels for over 25 years. She is also a program evaluator with the Accreditation Commission for Education in Nursing, Inc.

Glenise McKenzie, PhD, RN, is a faculty member at Oregon Health and Science University, Portland, OR. Glenise has over 25 years of clinical experience in the areas of mental health and gerontology. She is passionate about promoting and maintaining the mental health of older adults and their caregivers. She is currently participating in two educational research grants: one as a member of the Oregon Geriatric Education Center grant team, and another as a co-investigator exploring the impact of simulation on student nurses' knowledge, attitude, and empathy related to individuals with severe mental illness through an NLN research grant.

Patricia McKnight, MSN, RN, is a nurse educator at the Clearfield County Career and Technology Center, Clearfield, PA, and previously taught at the Cass Career Center, Harrisonville, MO. Patricia has been educating practical nurses for the past 15 years and has worked in many areas within the field of nursing during her career.

Sharon Elizabeth Metcalfe, EdD, RN, is currently an associate professor of nursing at Western Carolina University in Asheville, NC. For over 8 years, Sharon has been an associate professor of nursing and has had previous academic appointments as a dean of nursing for a private and community college. Additionally, she has been an educational grants researcher and has focused on grant funding for partnerships with colleges and medical facilities. Sharon also serves on the board of the North Carolina Nursing Association Foundation.

Heidi M. Meyer, MSN, RN, PHN, is an assistant professor of nursing at Gustavus Adolphus College, St. Peter, MN. As part of the Minnesota Intercollegiate Nursing Consortium (MINC), her primary teaching responsibilities include health assessment and adult health medical-surgical nursing. Her research interests include technology in nursing education, simulation in nursing education, and public health nursing.

Kerry A. Milner, DNSc, RN, is an assistant professor of nursing at Sacred Heart University School of Nursing, Fairfield, CT. For the past 3 years, Kerry has been teaching undergraduate and doctoral students about evidence-based practice, research methods, and biostatistics. She assisted with the accreditation process of the new DNP program at Sacred Heart University. Her research interests include gender, racial, and age differences in cardiovascular disease.

Sue Naumes, MSN, RN, has been practicing nursing in southern Oregon for over 30 years in a variety of settings, including 20 years as an instructor in the associate degree nursing program at the Rogue Community College (RCC) in Grants Pass, OR. As the program's clinical coordinator, Sue has developed many acute-care and nonacute-care clinical learning opportunities, including all concept-based clinical learning activities. Sue is also actively engaged in the Oregon Consortium for Nursing Education Research and Evaluation Committee.

Joanne Noone, PhD, RN, CNE, is an associate professor and campus associate dean at Oregon Health and Science University, Ashland, OR. Joanne has over 25 years of teaching nursing, in associate degree and baccalaureate programs, RN to BS completion programs, as well as master's and doctoral programs. Joanne's interests include health equity, cultural competence, and nursing workforce diversity. She received grant funding from the Oregon Center for Nursing Nurturing Cultural Competence in Nursing initiative to develop cultural competence learning activities.

Patty M. Orr, EdD, RN, is the director and chair of excellence at Austin Peay State University School of Nursing, Clarksville, TN. She has 17 years of teaching experience in associate, baccalaureate, and MSN nursing programs. For 20 years she served as a senior vice-president of a health care company that provides preventative and population health and disease management clinical services for participants of health plans and/or employers. Patty presently has four community-based grants that provide opportunities for BSN students to provide prevention and disease management for the underserved population in middle Tennessee.

Karen J. Polvado, DNP, RN, FNP-BC, is chair and associate professor of the Wilson School of Nursing at Midwestern State University, Wichita Falls, TX. Karen has an established record of program development, curriculum design/revision, and evaluation. Karen has a history of initiatives focused on student retention and success, many of which have been grant funded. Karen is committed to ensuring that nursing graduates, undergraduate and graduate, are prepared to face the challenges of an evolving health care environment.

Richard L. Pullen, Jr., EdD, RN, CMSRN, is the assistant director of the associate degree nursing program at Amarillo College, Amarillo, TX, and has served there for 20 years as a professor of nursing. His research and writing interests include nutrition, autoimmune disease, Socratic learning, models that promote student success, and faculty mentoring. He is the author of the care group model and end-of-life care interdisciplinary team clinical simulation model.

Kimberly H. Raines, PhD, CRNP, has been an RN since 1985 and a women's health nurse practitioner since 1997. Shes has a doctorate in adult education and has been teaching nursing for 12 years. Currently, she teaches in the American Public University System's RN-to-BSN program based in Charles Town, WV.

Alice Raymond, PhD, RN-BC, is the director of institutional effectiveness/Title III administrator at J. F. Drake State Technical College in Huntsville, AL. Alice has over 29 years of experience as a nurse, educator, and administrator. She has served as an educator in a health care facility, and has served as a nursing instructor and chairperson of its health sciences division. In her current role, she is responsible for institutional research, and maintaining institutional and programmatic accreditation.

Monique Ridosh, MSN, RN, is the director of the RN-to-BSN program and instructor in the Niehoff School of Nursing at Loyola University Chicago and PhD candidate at University of Wisconsin–Milwaukee. She teaches nursing undergraduates, designed the RN-to-BSN online courses, and is responsible for ongoing program development of the RN-to-BSN track. Over the past 18 years as a nurse, her clinical practice expertise is in pediatric nursing and her research interest is to understand experiences of families with children with chronic health conditions. Monique is an expert in online teaching methodologies and is a certified online educator at Loyola University Chicago.

Lori Rodriguez, PhD, RN, CNE, FNP, is an associate professor at The Valley Foundation School of Nursing at San Jose State University. She is the co-director of the California State University, Northern California Consortium DNP program. For over 30 years, Lori has been focused on the development of both undergraduate and graduate nurses in academia and hospital settings.

Kristen A. Sethares, PhD, RN, CNE, is an associate professor of nursing at the University of Massachusetts–Dartmouth, where she has taught students at all program levels for over 16 years. Kristen's area of research interest is heart failure self-care and patient decision making, especially concerning symptom management. She served as chair of the American Heart Association Nursing Education Committee in Massachusetts, on the Nursing Committee of the Heart Failure Society of America (2005–2011), and the Research Committee of the American Association of Heart Failure Nurses.

Lyndi C. Shadbolt, MS, RN, is an associate professor of nursing at Amarillo College, Amarillo, TX. She began her career in nursing education in 1995, teaching in all areas of the vocational nursing program. In 2006, she transitioned to the associate degree nursing program and continues to teach there in the classroom and clinical areas. Her areas of specialization include pharmacology, medical-surgical, and obstetrics.

Stephanie Sideras, PhD, RN, is an assistant professor at Oregon Health and Science University School of Nursing at the Ashland campus. She has been immersed in teaching with simulation since 2005. Her simulation philosophy emphasizes providing a high level of fidelity in order to augment the clinical setting. She has developed simulations that are carefully crafted in terms of setting, scripting, and technology interface to coach students though a patient care situation from start to finish rather than a single "snapshot" approach. Her doctoral work focused on evaluation of student clinical judgment in simulation, which continues to be her passion in her ongoing research.

Phyllis Ann Solari-Twadell, PhD, RN, FAAN, is an associate professor, tenured in the Niehoff School of Nursing, at Loyola University Chicago. She was employed for 25 years at Advocate Health Care in Park Ridge, IL. For the last 15 of the 25 years, Ann was director of The International Parish Nurse Resource Center, Advocate Health Care, Park Ridge. In that capacity, she was the editor of *Perspectives on Parish Nursing Practice*. Ann also coordinated 15 annual Granger Westberg Symposium on parish nursing and the development of a standardized core curriculum for parish nurses. Ann has co-edited and is a contributing author of the text *Parish Nursing: The Developing Practice, Parish Nursing: Promoting Whole Person Health within Faith Communities* and *Parish Nursing: Development, Education and Administration.*

Shirlee J. Snyder, EdD, RN, has been involved in nursing education as a faculty member and dean/director for over 35 years at Nevada State College, Henderson, NV. She has participated in practical nursing, associate degree, baccalaureate, and graduate nursing programs. Shirlee has served as a site visitor and evaluator for the Northwest Association of Schools and Colleges (NWASC) and the National League for Nursing Accrediting Commission (NLNAC). She is co-author of Kozier and Erb's *Fundamentals of Nursing and Skills in Clinical Nursing.*

Sandra M. Swoboda, MS, RN, FCCM, is a leader of the simulation team at Johns Hopkins University School of Nursing. She was the co-coordinator of the National Council of State Boards of Nursing (NCSBN) simulation study at the school and has over 15 years of experience as an educator, lecturer, and mentor in the clinical education setting. She has 19 years of clinical trial experience and has served as a senior research program coordinator in the Department of Surgery at the School of Medicine, in charge of all aspects of clinical trials in the surgical intensive care unit, including multicenter pharmaceutical-sponsored trials and site investigator/self-initiated studies. As a surgical critical care nurse, she continues to provide bedside care and serve in a leadership capacity to the staff.

Heather Voss, MSN, RN, clinical assistant professor, teaches population-based care and leadership in the undergraduate nursing program at Oregon Health and Science University, Ashland, OR. Heather collaborates with community partners to create authentic learning experiences for nursing students. She currently serves as president of the Beta Psi chapter, Sigma Theta Tau International.

Beth A. Vottero, PhD, RN, CNE, is an assistant professor of nursing at Purdue University Calumet in Hammond, IN and research associate with the Indiana Center for Evidence-Based Nursing Practice, a Joanna Briggs Institute collaborating center. Prior to moving into academia, Beth worked for 15 years as a staff and charge nurse on an intermediate care unit before becoming a magnet program director, spearheading the successful magnet redesignation of Indiana University Health La Porte Hospital. The experience helped focus her current research agenda on medication errors resulting from interruptions and distractions, for which she has received grant funding.

Kathleen B. Wilson, MSN, RN, CNE, is a senior instructor and online RN-to-BSN coordinator in the College of Nursing and Allied Health Professions at the University of Louisiana at Lafayette. Kathleen has been a classroom and clinical instructor in the College of Nursing for five years. Her nursing experience also includes medical-surgical nursing, intensive care nursing, risk management within a hospital, and serving as chief nursing officer in a nursing home.

Carolyn B. Yucha, PhD, RN, FAAN, is dean of the Schools of Nursing and Allied Health Sciences at the University of Nevada, Las Vegas. She was a developer of the Clinical Simulation Center of Las Vegas and serves on its advisory committee. She earned her PhD in physiology from Upstate Medical Center, Syracuse, NY. Carolyn has received research funding from the National Institutes of Health, has published numerous articles, and is editor of a scientific journal, *Biological Research for Nursing.*

Foreword

The evidence-based recommendations in the landmark Institute of Medicine (IOM) report, *The Future of Nursing: Leading Change, Advancing Health*, offer a blueprint for strengthening nursing education to ensure that nurses are prepared to take on more complex roles to meet our nation's current and future health demands. We must rise to the occasion! Our country needs nurses with strong clinical and leadership skills to help promote wellness, develop new models of care, manage care coordination, and help hospitals to reduce medical errors and rehospitalizations. That's why the IOM report calls for nurses to achieve higher levels of education and training through an innovative education system that promotes seamless academic progression.

In fact, strengthening nursing education is key to implementing the IOM report recommendations: the report's vision of nurses leading change and advancing health will only be fully realized if nursing faculty members are willing to embrace substantial changes to the nursing curricula, promote academic progression, and form unprecedented partnerships with leaders in practice that fully prepare nurses to take on more complex roles in the hospital, home, and community. Fortunately, as I travel the country in my role as the director of *The Future of Nursing: Campaign for Action,* a joint initiative of the Robert Wood Johnson Foundation and the AARP to help to implement the IOM recommendations, I am humbled and awed by the countless academic nurse leaders at community colleges and research universities alike who are transforming nursing education in their classrooms and communities to meet our country's changing health care needs. These leaders are part of a cadre of professionals who exemplify what the authors of the IOM report envisioned with its recommendation that nursing education programs and nursing associations prepare and enable nurses to lead change to advance health.

The National League for Nursing captures these leaders and their innovations in a prescient book, *Innovations in Nursing Education: Building the Future of Nursing,* which showcases how faculty at all levels of nursing education are strengthening education by emphasizing quality and safety in classrooms, fostering partnerships, teaching critical-thinking skills, and advancing academic progression. This book offers learning strategies that faculty throughout the country can adopt to ensure that our country succeeds in implementing the IOM recommendations and, ultimately, in building a strong and diverse workforce that advances our nation's health. I commend the National League for Nursing for featuring the best that nursing education has to offer and making it accessible to nursing faculty leaders to use in their classrooms.

Susan B. Hassmiller, PhD, RN, FAAN
Robert Wood Johnson Foundation
Senior Adviser for Nursing
Director, Future of Nursing: Campaign
for Action

Preface

The mission of the National League for Nursing (NLN) is to promote excellence in nursing education to build a strong and diverse nursing workforce to advance the nation's health. NLN efforts to fulfill this mission are based on four core values: caring, integrity, diversity, and excellence. Although all four values are expressed in this book, the primary focus is on excellence. According to the NLN: "A culture of excellence reflects a commitment to continuous growth, improvement, and understanding. It is a culture where transformation is embraced, and the status quo and mediocrity are not tolerated."

With this book, the NLN mission and core value of excellence are linked to the work of the Institute of Medicine (IOM) as reported in *The Future of Nursing: Leading Change, Advancing Health,* and in *A Summary of the February 2010 Forum on the Future of Nursing.* The IOM's publication provides direction for nursing practice, nursing leadership, and nursing education. These works by the IOM serve as a point of reference for this collection of peer-reviewed articles, accepted originally for publication in the Innovation Center of the NLN research journal, *Nursing Education Perspectives.* Each article showcases how faculty at all levels of nursing education, nationally and internationally, are implementing the recommendations of the *Future of Nursing* report. Many, many excellent faculty in schools of nursing are implementing these recommendations on a daily basis in numerous, often seemingly small ways. Yet these small ways are the building blocks that will lead to a future of excellence in nursing education.

The NLN is proud to present these innovative teaching/learning strategies as we work toward a bright future for nursing. We encourage all readers to consider sharing their day-to-day expressions of excellence with their nursing colleagues. As we all work together, excellence in nursing education becomes not a recommendation but a reality.

Linda Caputi, EdD, RN, CNE, ANEF
Professor Emerita of Nursing
College of DuPage
Glen Ellyn, Illinois
President, Linda Caputi, Inc.
Saint Charles, Illinois
Editor, Innovation Center,
Nursing Education Perspectives

References

Institute of Medicine (IOM). (2010). *A summary of the February 2010 forum on the future of nursing.* Washington, DC: National Academies Press.

Institute of Medicine (IOM). (2011). *The future of nursing: Leading change, advancing health.* Washington, DC: National Academies Press.

Contents

List of Figures and Tables

LIST OF TABLES

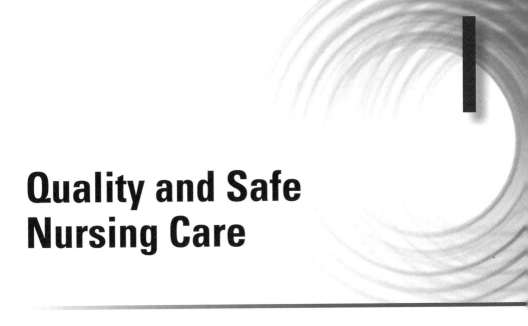

Quality and Safe Nursing Care

References to quality and safety concepts are present throughout the Institute of Medicine's 2011 report, *The Future of Nursing: Leading Change, Advancing Health*. The report contains the following:

- Chapter 2, "Study Context," specifically addresses quality and the quality improvement movement, patient-centered care, and interprofessional collaboration.
- Chapter 3, "Transforming Practice," continues the discussion of patient-centered care and interprofessional collaboration, along with a focus on the importance of higher-quality care, safety, and informatics.
- Chapter 5, "Transforming Leadership," discusses the need for more nurse researchers to expand the evidence base for nursing care and improved models of care.

These same concepts are addressed throughout *A Summary of the February 2010 Forum on the Future of Nursing* as major areas of concern in curricula preparing both entry-level nursing professionals and advanced practice nurses (APNs). With their incorporation into the learning outcomes of most schools of nursing, these concepts are becoming a standard part of nursing curricula.

In this section, Chapters 1 through 7 present innovative methods and educational environments for incorporating these concepts into the practice of nurse educators as they prepare their nursing graduates to provide safe, evidence-based, quality care in their current practice and throughout their careers.

Reference

Institute of Medicine. (2011). *The future of nursing: Leading change, advancing health*. Washington, DC: The National Academies Press.

Applying Safety in the Clinical Setting: Teaching Students the Significance of Clinical Alarms

Katherine B. Ardoin, MSN, RN, CNE
Kathleen B. Wilson, MSN, RN, CNE

The Joint Commission and the American College of Clinical Engineering (ACCE, 2006; HCPro, 2005) are placing increased emphasis on alarm safety in the clinical setting. HCPro noted that the Joint Commission has included alarm safety within its accreditation standards, while the ACCE has published a White Paper focusing on clinical alarm issues (ACCE, 2006; HCPro, 2005). These publications assert that nursing graduates have the same problems as experienced nurses with perceiving an alarm sound as an alert to a patient issue that needs attention.

The Quality and Safety Education for Nurses (QSEN) Institute (www.qsen.org) is concerned about the quality and safety gap between the learning environment and practice setting (Thornlow & McGuinn, 2010). The American Association of Colleges of Nursing (AACN) integrated QSEN's recommendations in its 2008 revision of the *Essentials of Baccalaureate Education for Professional Nursing Practice.* No longer can quality and safety in patient care be merely an underlying theme in undergraduate nursing education; rather, it must be a focus of the expected outcomes for graduates of a nursing program.

An opportune time for nursing instructors to initiate attention to alarms is during clinical instruction. QSEN offers informative resources for nursing instructors to learn how to implement quality and safety educational tools to advance the knowledge and skills of nursing students (Thornlow & McGuinn, 2010). We chose one of these QSEN clinical teaching strategies to introduce our students to alarm safety and increase students' awareness of clinical alarms to facilitate assimilation of quality and safety values in patient care.

SETTING THE STAGE

Clinical alarms have been a mainstay in the health care setting as alerts that a device or person needs attention. Alarms help diagnose, treat, or monitor via audible and/or visual warnings when a patient's physiologic parameter(s) has surpassed the preset limits. Alarms also serve to warn clinicians of an actual or imminent equipment failure (Phillips, 2006). Alarm classifications present as true and clinically relevant, true and clinically irrelevant, or false (nuisance).

- *True and clinically relevant* alarms send notifications when clinical changes require an intervention, such as when a patient's oxygen saturation falls below 95 percent despite inactivity (Phillips, 2006).

- An alarm is *true and clinically irrelevant* when the parameter will reset to baseline without treatment, as when a patient's oxygen saturation falls below 95 percent while being suctioned (Phillips, 2006).

- A *false (nuisance)* alarm occurs when the alarm parameters are breached; however, the breach is not part of the clinical picture (Phillips, 2006). False alarms might occur when a patient's typical oxygen saturation is 93 percent and the monitor alarms for drops below 95 percent.

When mistakes concerning alarm safety in the clinical setting happen, the cause is generally an individual performance issue and/or a system effectiveness concern (QSEN, 2011). Either the alarm fails to capture the clinician's attention, or a mechanical, environmental, or user problem leads to a breach in patient safety.

Employee attentiveness is a critical factor in alarm safety. Being attentive to sounding alarms means that the clinician is able to filter out irrelevant information while fully processing and perceiving the relevant stimulus (Curry, Meyers, & McKinney, 2006; Green, 2009). Inattentional blindness (IB) occurs when an individual is unaware of an unexpected (salient) stimulus because attention is focused on another task or item (Mack & Roche, 1998 as cited Karns & Rivardo, 2010). The cause is not carelessness or lack of common sense; rather it is a natural human occurrence of limited mental attention combined with high adaptability (Green, 2009). Although much research regarding attentiveness to stimuli and prevention of accidents includes visual perception, Curry et al. (2006) described a case in which IB involved auditory senses of workers painting a high-intensity radio transmission antenna on a large building. Due to multiple false alarms (transient radio transmissions requiring frequent resetting) the painters dismissed warning information about a true condition.

Cognitive conspicuity, or the ability to identify relevance of information, is one way of explaining how and when a person pays attention to a stimulus ("Inattentional Blindness," 2009). For example, while on the way to a patient's room to respond to an intravenous (IV) pump alarm, the nurse hears a second IV pump alarm from another room. Something triggers the nurse to decide that the first alarm is more important. Because sensing and perceiving happen so quickly, sometimes attention divides and people sense the sound, but do not perceive the meaning in the same way (Green, 2009). Here, the nurse placed higher relevance on the first alarm due to the nature of the medication infusing.

Mental workload and task interference (multitasking) is a second explanation for how and when a person attends to stimuli, especially those stimuli involving the same senses at the same time, such as listening to two equally important but different alarms simultaneously ("Inattentional Blindness," 2009). For instance, the nurse hears an IV pump and an enteral tube-feeding pump alarm concurrently for the same patient. While the nurse is responding to the alarm of one pump, the second pump alarm distracts part of the nurse's attention, causing a misstep in reprogramming the first pump, and thus a mistake in treatment.

Past experiences and counterintuitiveness are a third explanation for attentiveness concerns. An experienced nurse who generally performs on instinct may not investigate all options (counter to what needs to happen) and, consequently, not notice the "real" problem (Curry et al., 2006; Green, 2009). For example, an experienced nurse reprograms an IV pump to silence a distal occlusion alarm without assessing the patient for a blood return, thereby failing to determine the presence of an infiltration.

The capacity to pay attention varies among individuals and often depends on their age and mental ability. Fatigue, distraction, and the sheer number of alarms (some of which are false) can compound the situation ("Inattentional Blindness," 2009). McKinney (2010) cited an incident involving nurses on a surgical floor who were no longer sensitive to a cardiac monitor alarm that was repeatedly sounding. The nurses did not report the repeated warning alarms and turned the volume on the bedside crisis alarm off, resulting in the death of a patient (McKinney, 2010).

A breach in patient safety can also arise from mechanical conditions, the working environment, or the user's technical abilities:

- Mechanical conditions can involve errors (e.g., equipment malfunction) or design flaw (e.g., generic preset parameters, oversensitive equipment sensors; ACCE, 2006).

- The working environment can contribute to breaches in patient safety due to the physical layout of workspaces or an increased patient-to-nurse ratio, either of which may place the nurse out of hearing range.

- Problems with the user's technical abilities include: improper selection, placement, or maintenance of IV lines, blood pressure cuffs, EKG leads, and oxygen sensors; incorrect setting of alarm parameters; and failure to turn alarms on. All can lead to a breach in patient safety (Bell, 2008; Green, 2009).

LEARNING ACTIVITY

The Alarm Safety Learning Activity

To help close the knowledge gap regarding quality and safety issues related to clinical alarms, we chose to implement the Alarm Safety Learning Activity, developed by Spencer and Fosse (2009), and available on the QSEN website (www.qsen.org/teachingstrategy. php?id=79). As part of the Alarm Safety Learning Activity, students complete a problem-based learning assignment while working on the clinical unit. At the end of the clinical day, the students answer reflective practice questions during postclinical conference and evaluation. The activity addresses the delivery of safe and effective care related to clinical alarms, and promotes collaboration, analysis, and interpretation of various roles of an interdisciplinary health care team. Instructors address individual performance related to clinical alarm safety and attend to system effectiveness through guided postactivity discussion questions (QSEN, 2011).

QSEN (2011) has proposed targets for the knowledge, skills, and attitudes for nursing prelicensure programs directed toward safety. The Alarm Safety Learning Activity addresses:

1. Knowledge—recognizing safety-enhancing technologies such as automatic alerts/alarms
2. Skills—the ability to demonstrate effective use of technology, implement strategies to reduce risk of harm, communicate observations or concerns related to hazards, analyze errors and design system improvements
3. Attitudes—valuing one's own role in preventing errors; valuing vigilance and monitoring performance of care by patients, families, and other members of the health care team (QSEN, 2011)

Spencer and Fosse (2009) recommend delaying the activity until students are self-directed in providing basic care for their patients and are open to begin recognizing, interpreting, and responding to clinical alarms. Students should also evaluate the activity with respect to what they learned, how the response is a nursing/health concern, who should answer the alarms, and whether they found the activity beneficial (Spencer & Fosse, 2009).

Implementation of the Alarm Safety Learning Activity

At semester midterm, a clinical group of first-semester junior nursing students demonstrated readiness to engage in a supplementary learning activity. Although Spencer and Fosse (2009) recommend administering the activity over one clinical day, we added an additional day to overcome the typical hectic pace of the first day of a new clinical week and to afford students the opportunity to attend to a greater variety of clinical alarms.

In preconference, the clinical instructor distributed to the students the Alarm Safety Learning Activity worksheet as well as brief instructions for its use. The students were to collect information consisting of the location and type of alarm, analyze possible alarm triggers, track who responded to the alarm, and determine what intervention the clinician performed in responding to the alarm. As students gathered data, they asked questions of nurses and their instructor, particularly if they were unfamiliar with a specific alarm. Students especially focused on IV pump alarms. On occasion, students coached each other through the troubleshooting messages, which increased their knowledge and skills regarding pump safety. Soon, students were answering IV pump alarms for nearly every patient on the unit, showing an increased proficiency attitude in their role of caring for patients with IV pumps.

Activity Outcomes

Postclinical conference was a time to reflect on the day's events regarding the alarm safety activity. Along with their answers to questions on the worksheet, students discussed various influences on clinical responses to alarms. Replying to the question, "Why are alarms ignored?" one student said, "Some nurses were not in close earshot of the alarms [work environment]." Another student responded, "Nurses might already know what the alarm meant, that it was not an emergency, and they would get to it shortly [cognitive conspicuity]." A third student answered, "Nurses were too busy to respond to other nurses' clinical alarms [capacity to pay attention]."

The next inquiry was, "What are nuisance alarms?" One student presented an example of an alarm sounding for a sequential compression device because it could not meet the set air-fill parameters; the patient was not wearing the device at the time.

In response to the question, "How would [you] reply to a patient's questions about an alarm?," students visualized themselves as a patient with an alarm sounding and no one coming, or taking a very long time, as well as how they might feel if the nurse did not take the alarm seriously. Stepping into the patient role was a revelation for them.

The final questions centered on prioritizing alarms on the clinical unit. The criteria included determining the seriousness of the patient's condition, identifying the physiological parameter the equipment was monitoring, and decoding the alarm prompt message. The clinical instructor asked students what tasks in answering the alarm they might delegate, what the nurse must do to satisfy the alarm message, and what assistance from a specially trained person might be required if unable to resolve the alarm. Students quickly identified alarms related to airway and breathing as the top priority for immediate intervention.

Students evaluated the clinical alarm safety activity in their weekly clinical journals. Comments of interest included:

- "Even if it's just an IV machine, you never know what the problem could be, and it can aggravate the patient [skills/attitudes]."
- "Sharing the reasons and interventions to the alarms we heard helped me to be more aware and effective in investigating the sound [knowledge]."
- "I found this discussion particularly helpful with prioritizing various alarms. It reminded me that alarms should not be ignored [knowledge]."
- "It made me realize I was tuning out alarms to some extent. I need to notice alarms and know what they signify [capacity to pay attention]."
- "I listened to alarms all day and discovered that they go off quite often [capacity to pay attention]."
- "It's clearer now that if I'm free to check on another patient, it could be beneficial to the patient and the nurse [capacity to pay attention]."

CONCLUSION

The ACCE White Paper (2006) revealed that graduating nurses have the same problems as experienced nurses in perceiving the sound of clinical alarms as important. We focused on student awareness of clinical alarms by implementing Spencer and Fosse's Alarm Safety Learning Activity (2009). The student responses during the postclinical conference and in their journals revealed they were beginning to internalize new values related to alarm recognition and safety. Student comments and actions illustrate that the activity met the QSEN (2011) proposed targets for knowledge, skills, and attitudes. Students demonstrated knowledge of safety-enhancing technologies by sharing reasons for answering clinical alarms and interventions taken in response to those alarms. They demonstrated effective use of technology by teaching each other how to troubleshoot alarms. Student comments illustrated awareness of the value of being attentive to clinical alarms and the need to act promptly to alarm sounds to foster a culture of caring for patients.

Although one clinical group responded appropriately to clinical alarm situations after the learning activity, a before-and-after research design with all students in the class will provide a better perspective on whether the learning activity raised the level of awareness of clinical alarms to promote assimilation of quality and safety values in student practice. It is our intent that the change in knowledge, skills, and attitudes related to alarm safety will lead to a change in practice by the students before and after graduation.

References

American College of Clinical Engineering (ACCE), Task Force on the Impact of Clinical Alarms in Patient Safety. (2006). White Pages of the ACCE on the Impact of Clinical Alarms on Patient Safety. ACCE Healthcare Technology Foundation. Plymouth Meeting, PA. Retrieved from www.acce-htf.org

Bell, L. (2008). Monitoring clinical alarms. *American Journal of Critical Care, 17*(1), 4.

Curry, D. G., Meyers, E., & McKinney, M. (2006). Seeing versus perceiving: What you see isn't always what you get. *Professional Safety, 51*(6), 28–34.

Green, M. (2009). Nursing error. Retrieved from http://www.visualexpert.com/Resources/nursingerror.html

HCPro. (2005). Why can't I find improving the effectiveness of clinical alarms on the list of National Patient Safety Goals? Retrieved from www.hcpro.com/ACC-44860-851/Why-can't-I-find-improving-the-effectiveness-of-clinical-alarms-in-the-list-of-National-Patient-Safety-Goals.html

Inattentional blindness: What captures your attention? (2009, February). Institute for Safe Medication Practices. Retrieved from www.ismp.org/newsletters/acutecare/articles/20090226.asp

Karns, T. C., & Rivardo, M. G. (2010). Noticing of an unexpected event is affected by attentional set for expected action. *North American Journal of Psychology, 12*(3), 637–650.

McKinney, M. (2010). Alarm fatigue sets off bells: Mass incident highlights needs for protocols check. *Modern Healthcare, 40*(15), 14.

Phillips, J. (2006). Clinical alarms: Complexity and common sense. *Critical Care Nursing Clinics of North America, 18*(2), 145–156. doi:10.1016/j.ccell.2006.01.002

Quality & Safety Education for Nurses (QSEN). (2011). Competency KSAs (prelicensure). Retrieved from http://qsen.org/ksas_prelicensure.php

Spencer, T., & Fosse, K. (2009). Alarm safety learning activity. *Quality & Safety Education for Nurses.* Retrieved from www.qsen.org/teachingstrategy.php?id=79

Thornlow, D. K., & McGuinn, K. (2010). A necessary sea of change for faculty development: Spotlight on quality and safety. *Journal of Professional Nursing, 21*(2), 71–81. doi: 10.1016/j.profnurs.2009.10.009.

Immersion into a Root Cause Analysis

Beth A. Vottero, PhD, RN, CNE

Teaching quality concepts in a nursing program poses unique challenges for nurse educators. A distinct need exists to infuse programs with quality concepts that encourage future nurses to practice accountability and responsibility, not only to their patients, but also to the nursing profession. The American Association of Colleges of Nursing (AACN) recognizes this need and promotes it through *Essential II: Basic Organizational and Systems Leadership for Patient Safety and Quality Care* (2009). In that initiative, the AACN (2009) recommends that nursing students learn to:

- Conduct a mock Root Cause Analysis (RCA) on a near miss and share results with staff or shared governance council.
- Participate in an actual RCA and/or Failure Mode Effects Analysis (FMEA).

Quality and Safety Education for Nursing (QSEN, 2011) is a related initiative that promotes quality knowledge, skills, and attitudes for prelicensure nurses. QSEN specifically calls for the following educational practices:

- Engage in an RCA rather than blaming when errors or near misses occur.
- Describe processes (such as RCA and FMEA) used in understanding causes of error and allocation of responsibility and accountability.

Involving students in an RCA and engaging them in each aspect of the steps promotes an understanding of the depth and breadth of unintentional health care errors. Immersing students in an RCA allows educators to focus on key learning outcomes such as focusing on process versus individual problems, responsibility and accountability to the profession of nursing, and how to define and measure quality outcomes. Replicating the RCA process using a systematic step-by-step process provides students opportunities to understand how the complex care environment can contribute to process breakdowns, resulting in unintentional errors.

An RCA is a systematic review of processes conducted when a sentinel event occurs. "A sentinel event is an unexpected occurrence that results in serious physical or psychological injury, death, or the risk thereof" (The Joint Commission, 2011, para. 1). The intent of an RCA is to develop an understanding of the underlying problems contributing to practice errors—understanding that focuses on process rather than individuals. In the RCA process, nurses must participate to provide the "voice" of the nurse not only in identifying problems, but also in developing solutions.

Based on the recommendations of the AACN and QSEN, nursing programs need to review their curricula for appropriate placement of a mock RCA.

DEVELOPMENT OF THE LESSON

At a midwestern university, the faculty identified Management and Leadership courses, clinical courses, or capstone preparation as possible venues for appropriate placement of a mock RCA. Faculty selected the capstone preparation course, a one-credit-hour didactic course that prepares students for the senior level capstone course, in which they complete a project that develops an evidence-based solution for a quality issue at an actual health care organization.

Within that capstone preparation course, the quality lesson is designed to follow the structure of an RCA as described by the Institute for Healthcare Improvement (Huber & Ogrinc, 2011). A packet is distributed to students describing an RCA and a sentinel event; the packet also defines the five steps of the RCA process (Box 2.1). In addition,

BOX 2.1 ROOT CAUSE ANALYSIS ROADMAP

Definitions

Root Cause Analysis (RCA): A systematic questioning process to identify the causal factors of an error or a near miss (The Joint Commission, 2011). An RCA is used to understand and prevent sentinel events. The process assumes that errors are a system failure rather than an individual mistake.

Sentinel event: Unexpected occurrence involving death or serious physical or psychological injury, or the risk thereof.

Focus: What happened? Why did it happen? How can we prevent it from happening again?

Step I: Gather Facts and Put Together a Team
1. Review documents related to the incident (medical records, incident reports, etc.).
2. Interview those involved and observe the "typical" process.
3. The team should:
   a. Be interdisciplinary
   b. Encompass all staff directly involved with the event
   c. Include administrative support staff

Step II: Understand What Happened
1. Review the timeline of events from each perspective.
2. Compare actual with best practice.
3. Begin to identify opportunities or ideas.

BOX 2.1 (continued)

Step III: Determine the Root Cause
1. Based on analysis of process, ask why, why, why, why, why (five times).
2. Create a fishbone diagram (Fig. 2.1) using the seven types of factors influencing errors.
   a. **Patient characteristics:** unique mix of factors that the patient presents. Physical condition, language preference, communication needs and barriers, social environment.
   b. **Task factors:** aspects of clinical tasks that make them safer or less safe. Protocols, clinical rules, design of tasks or structure, how information is used and transmitted, including test results.
   c. **Individual staff member:** how staff members influence safety. Knowledge, skills, motivation, and health of practitioners involved in care.
   d. **Team factors:** all the ways that people work together. Communication, explicit or implicit hierarchies, responsiveness of supervisors, ease with which team members ask for help and clarification.
   e. **Work environment:** working conditions. Where we work influences how we work. Staffing levels, workload, levels of experience, equipment, and administrative support.
   f. **Organizational and management factors:** values of the health care organization translate into clinical practice. Do standards and policies support safety? Is culture patient centered or provider centered? Severe financial constraints? Culture of safety versus culture of blame?
   g. **Institutional context:** external environment in which the hospital sits. Includes state and national regulations, financial and economic factors, shareholders or taxpayers who support the hospital.
3. Identify "contributing" causes (if fixed, would help but not prevent problem).
4. Identify "root" causes (if fixed, would prevent the problem).

Step IV: Establish a Risk Reduction Plan
1. For each cause, identify corrective measures and improvement opportunities.
2. Create a timeline and assign responsibilities.

Step V: Evaluate Effectiveness of Plan
1. Report back to team with findings, changes, outcomes, data (if possible).

SOURCE: Adapted from Institute for Healthcare Improvement (Huber & Ogrinc, 2011).

students are given the patient assessment, the Medication Administration Record, physician order sheets, a risk reduction plan table, and change proposal. The packet mimics actual practice, in which all participants in the RCA are given access to records relating to the event. The information in the packet enables students to develop an understanding of the context in which the error occurred.

To immerse students in the RCA, the instructor initiates the class with a brief background of the incident by playing the role of the quality representative:

> We are here today because a 24-year-old man came to the ED seeking treatment for appendicitis at 10:30 AM. He was transferred to the Medical Unit at 1:00 PM after being seen by the physician and receiving orders. At 8:30 PM, he was found apneic and unresponsive in his bed. We need to identify what happened to this healthy male patient.

BOX 2.2 ROLE EXAMPLE: DAY SHIFT MEDICAL-SURGICAL NURSE

You received the patient, Mr. Jones, a 24 y/o male from the ED, at 1:00 PM with a medical diagnosis of appendicitis. He is 6'2" and 208 lbs. He received 2 mg morphine IVP in the ED at 11:45 AM with some relief. He still complains of pain and has a standing order for 1–2 mg morphine every 1–2 hours PRN for pain. He received another 2 mg morphine in the ED at 12:45 PM. Your charting shows the following:

1:30p: 2 mg morphine IVP for pain rating of 8. HR 108, BP 124/72, Resp 22.
1:45p: Patient states some pain relief. Pain now at 5.
2:30p: Patient states pain at 8. 2 mg morphine IVP given.
3:00p: Pain rated at 6. HR 122, BP 108/64, Resp 24.

Admission assessment: Completed while caring for four other high-acuity patients. You didn't have a lot of time to spend with Mr. Jones as another patient was experiencing chest pain and you just received a post-op colostomy patient at the same time.

Report given to evening shift nurse: You explained the problems controlling the pain. The patient is scheduled for surgery to remove the appendix in the morning and is NPO until after the procedure. Currently the patient is awake, alert, and oriented. No past medical history and no allergies. He works for the railroad as an engineer.

The following describes how the steps in an RCA are interpreted and operationalized for the classroom setting.

Step I: Gather Facts and Put Together a Team

The students are welcomed to the RCA committee meeting and brief role descriptions are distributed to select students (Box 2.2). Each description includes the team members' perspective, what they were thinking and doing during the time frame, and the intent of their actions. The roles include day shift and evening shift nurses on a medical-surgical unit, Emergency Department (ED) day shift nurse, medical-surgical unit charge nurse and unit director, physician, patient, patient's wife, pharmacist, and respiratory therapist.

The faculty initiates a conversation to determine which roles should be included on the team. The class discusses the roles and the pros and cons for inclusion of each. An essential part of the discussion is the need for a variety of perspectives from different role players. Students assume the assigned roles and are called upon during the RCA to present their sides of the story. The discussion covers the need for nurse participation in the RCA to provide the "voice" of the bedside nurse—a critical need when discussing any patient care issue. To encourage discussion, the instructor prompts sharing by students.

Step II: Understand What Happened

To fully comprehend the complexity of the problem, a timeline that starts when the patient entered the ED is constructed with student input. The students use the information from the packet to reconstruct what happened, including events such as medication dosing, assessments, and other relevant information. During this step, the instructor guides the students in identifying decision points and where breakdowns in the process occurred. The timeline is reviewed from each participant's perspective to develop a big-picture idea of what happened.

As students begin to identify where processes broke down, the instructor prompts them to think on a deeper level by asking why. Standard practice in identifying a true cause requires asking "why" five times (Huber & Ogrinc, 2011).

> The students quickly identify that the patient received multiple doses of a narcotic in a narrow timeframe. The first "why" query brings forth superficial responses that point the finger at the nurse, such as, "The nurse gave too many doses." The second time the students are asked why, they begin to move beyond the nurse. By the fourth time, students begin to see that there is a deeper cause for overuse of narcotics in this case. For example:
>
> - Why #1: Because the nurse gave too many doses
> - Why #2: Because the nurse did not see that a dose was given 15 minutes prior
> - Why #3: Because it wasn't documented
> - Why #4: Because the nurse covering for the first nurse didn't put it in the record
> - Why #5: Because when a narcotic is removed, it isn't automatically recorded

At this point, the instructor uses this opportunity to discuss how nurses are at the sharp end, where problems materialize due to deeper process issues (Hughes, 2008). The process problems align to create opportunities for failure. Students begin to see that the sentinel event is a result of deeper issues beyond the event in and of itself.

Each problem arising from the timeline construction activity is subjected to the "five why" questioning technique. This method initiates the process of "drilling down" into the core process failures that allowed the problem to occur. Thus, Step II promotes an understanding of what happened prior to the sentinel event and, in turn, allows for an exploration of potential causative factors. Identifying the true causes provides a *foundation for the next step.*

Step III: Determine the Root Cause

Step III involves creating a fishbone analysis of causative factors. The Agency for Healthcare Research and Quality's Patient Safety Network provides a list and examples of seven common causes that lead to latent errors (AHRQ, 2011). These seven causes become the "bones" of the fish, helping to organize facts from the scenario. Figure 2.1 shows how the fishbone looks after discussing one aspect of the scenario: medication dosing.

On a fishbone chart, participants can visually link the causes and the outcome. Student discussion involves identifying the root cause and creating a plan to fix the problem. For example, when discussing the timing of medication administration, the students identified two issues:

1. Handoff communication when staff took a break did not conform to regular end-of-shift handoffs in that it was a quick overview rather than a list of specific patient needs for the time frame of the break.

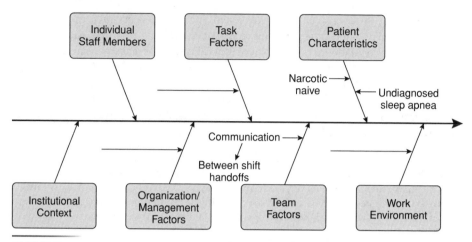

FIGURE 2.1 Fishbone analysis.

2. The electronic medication system did not stop the nurse from withdrawing a narcotic even though it was outside the boundaries of the dosing schedule. If the medication system had prevented removal of a dose, then the rapid dosing would not have occurred.

These two process problems become the focus for creating a risk reduction plan in Step IV.

Step IV: Establish a Risk Reduction Plan

The class identifies two issues: handoff communication for breaks and hard stops for withdrawing narcotics outside the dosing time frame. These issues form the basis for a risk-reduction plan. In this step, students take each issue and develop a risk-reduction plan for change. The plan includes the following components:

- Action item
- Risk-reduction strategies
- Measure of effectiveness
- Timeline
- Person responsible

To assist students in creating the risk-reduction plan, the instructor walks them through an example using hard stops for narcotic administration. The class then discusses potential risk-reduction strategies, exploring strategies that reduce the chance of recurrence and how each strategy's risk would be measured. The students identify the need to eliminate the opportunity of removing narcotic medications outside of the set time, and determine that reprogramming the electronic medication system to include a hard stop would prevent a similar error.

Measuring the effectiveness of any improvement project is a crucial step and provides an opportunity to dialogue with students about quality measures. In this particular lesson, in lieu of Step V (Evaluate Effectiveness of Plan), students identified desired outcomes and brainstormed ways to quantifiably measure outcomes. Discussion included a definition of indicators and benchmarks as well as quality information from the National Database of Nurse Sensitive Indicators, National Quality Forum, National Patient Safety Goals, and Healthy People 2020. By including quality indicators and benchmarks within the RCA, students developed an awareness and understanding of larger quality principles. Measuring the effectiveness of hard stops in electronic medication systems included monitoring pharmacy reports of attempts to withdraw narcotics, number of overrides to access narcotics, and number of rapid-response team calls related to oversedation.

The final part of the risk-reduction plan is creating a timeline and identification of persons responsible for implementing the change. The instructor reinforced the need to be specific so that all participants in the RCA knew exactly what they had to do and by when, eliminating redundancy and increasing efficiency. To illustrate this point, the instructor offered a short scenario about nurses lacking a time frame for completion and not knowing who was assigned what part of the task. Students were encouraged to contribute to the discussion with similar experiences. To complete the risk-reduction plan, the instructor stressed the need for including a nurse in any team created to address an issue involving patient care.

IMPLEMENTATION OF THE LESSON

To allow time for deeper understanding of material, Steps I, II, and III occurred during one class session and Steps IV and V followed at the next. Students were given a risk-reduction-plan table and guiding questions to complete between course meetings. The guiding questions required students to review the evidence on their issue to begin forming a new policy or procedure relevant to their problem. The students were also required to create a PICO (population, intervention, comparison, and outcome) question to guide their review of the literature.

Step V, Evaluate Effectiveness of Plan, included reporting back to the team with findings, changes, outcomes, and data. This was not completed in class but was included in the discussion. Reporting is an important element in communication: bringing actions completed back to the main group as well as disseminating information to larger hospital-wide committees or shared-governance councils.

CONCLUSION

This lesson provided students the opportunity to participate in an RCA—from identification of a problem through development of a risk-reduction plan. Students learned how to determine individual versus process problems by following the steps of the RCA, including how to drill down a problem to determine those factors contributing to the error. Throughout the lesson, a sense of accountability and responsibility to the nursing profession resulted from stressing nurse presence on any team created to address a patient care issue. Introducing the concepts of accountability and responsibility occurred both in Step I and Step IV. The final intent of the lesson involved how to define and measure quality outcomes. The content in Step IV covered quality measure sources and selection of appropriate measures of outcomes.

Course evaluations revealed that students enjoyed the experience, feeling that they had a better understanding of how multidisciplinary teams work together to support safe environments for patient care. A survey of students after the lesson found that 100 percent strongly agreed that it is important for nurses to be involved in an RCA. Asked about the lesson, 83 percent found it helped them to understand quality patient care measurements and outcomes. The survey included value questions and open-ended responses about the lesson, including the following:

- Why is it important to be a part of a root cause analysis?
- Did the root cause analysis lesson help you understand quality patient care measurements and outcomes?
- What did you like best about the RCA lesson?
- What could be done to improve the RCA lesson?

Student comments included:

- I liked looking at a situation from many different points of view, focusing on many different angles of the situation.
- I liked learning that it is important for the RN to be involved to aid in getting down to the point and making a change for the better.
- Collaboration of team member participation and critical thinking that it takes to find out what happened and how to prevent it from occurring again.
- How it taught us to not be scared of the RCA process and how it may look like the nurse's fault but a lot of times it is a group effort that caused the problem. I also liked how you used real-life stories.

Student responses demonstrate the achievement of intended learning outcomes. Suggestions for improving the lesson included creating movie clips on portions of the scenario and showing them during class, creating audio clips of the various perspectives from those involved in the sentinel event, and providing additional resources for nurses to protect themselves. Exploration of multimedia presentation methods are currently being reviewed for inclusion based on comments.

A need exists to not only evaluate the lesson and course, but also to investigate the sustainability of learning outside of the classroom. The transfer of learning from the classroom context into clinical practice is a desired outcome of all courses. Research is needed on the effect of the RCA lesson after graduation and employment as an RN.

References

Agency for Healthcare Research and Quality (AHRQ) Patient Safety Network. (2011). *Patient Safety Primers: Root Cause Analysis.* Retrieved from http://psnet.ahrq.gov/primer.aspx?primerID=10

American Association of Colleges of Nursing (AACN). (2009). *Nurse Faculty Toolkit for the Implementation of The Baccalaureate Essentials.* Retrieved from http://www.aacn.nche.edu/Education/pdf/BacEssToolkit.pdf

Huber, S., & Ogrinc, G. (2011). *Institute for Healthcare Improvement Course: Root cause and systems analysis.* Retrieved from http://app.ihi.org/lms/coursedetailview. aspx?CourseGUID=450435c3f015- 4541-943246eb235461bb&CatalogGUID=6 cb1c614-884b-43ef-9abdd90849f183d4

Hughes, R. (2008). *Patient Safety and Quality: An Evidence-Based Handbook for Nurses.* Volume 1. AHRQ Publication No. 08-0043. Agency for Healthcare Research and Quality, Rockville, MD. Retrieved from http://www.ahrq.gov/qual/nurseshdbk/

Quality & Safety Education for Nurses (QSEN). (2011). Competency KSAs [Knowledge, Skills, Attitudes]: Prelicensure. Retrieved from http://www.qsen.org/ksas_prelicensure.php

The Joint Commission. (2011). *Facts about the sentinel event policy.* Retrieved from http://www.jointcommission.org/assets/ 1/18/Sentinel_Event_Policy_3_2011.pdf

3

Health Literacy:
Demonstrating Achievement of the QSEN Competencies in a Senior Capstone Project

Lori Rodriguez, PhD, RN, CNE, FNP

This article describes a project for senior baccalaureate students that integrates an understanding of health literacy while achieving several quality and safety competencies. Limited health literacy directly affects patients' lives and the cost of health care. Teaching patients how to manage their own health and illness is an essential competency for nursing students (Cormier & Kotrlik, 2009).

Health literacy is the ability of the patient and/or caregiver to understand and apply basic health information and services to help the patient make good, safe decisions. Patients with low health literacy are at risk for poor health outcomes, health disparities, and low life expectancy (Sudore et al., 2009; Sudore, Mehta et al., 2006; Sudore, Yaffe et al., 2006). The National Patient Safety Foundation (2010) reports low health literacy skills as a stronger predictor of health status than the individual's age, income, employment status, education level, or racial/ethnic group. Limited health literacy can lead to higher rates of hospitalization, worsening of chronic medical conditions, and less use of preventative services.

In 2010, the American Nurses Association (ANA) House of Delegates approved a resolution emphasizing the importance of improving health literacy in the health care environment. This resolution stated the need for increased health literacy knowledge and skills in nursing school curricula (Trossman, 2010). To this end, a project was developed for senior nursing students that requires the integration and performance of multiple competencies to positively affect a patient's health literacy. The project's results also demonstrate a number of the Quality and Safety Education for Nurses (QSEN) competencies, including the following:

- Seeing the patient's illness "through the patient's eyes"
- Respecting and encouraging individual patient values and cultural preferences

- Providing patient care with sensitivity and respect
- Discussing principles of effective communication
- Improving patients' understanding of their disease and its management
- Recognizing the patient or designee as a source of control and full partner in coordinating the patient's or surrogate's needs by taking into account patient preferences, values, and needs

Students who completed this project were enthusiastic, stating that they could see the results of their efforts and how it makes a difference to the patient. As one student remarked, "Health literacy is the main underlying engine to effective patient teaching."

THE HEALTH LITERACY PROJECT

At the beginning of their final senior capstone semester, students participate in a one-hour conference in which the concept of health literacy is discussed. For most students, health literacy is not a new concept, but this conference asks them to integrate evidence about health literacy and the patient's condition, background, culture, language, reading ability, family dynamics, and other individual characteristics. They use this information to develop an activity with the goal of improving their patient's health literacy.

Most students engaged in patient teaching projects throughout nursing school. With this assignment the students must focus on the outcome of their teaching. A simple diagram is used to demonstrate to the students the difference between patient teaching, which is a nursing intervention, and health literacy, which is the desired patient outcome (Figure 3.1).

Students are asked to conduct a literature search on health literacy with a focus on the types of patients they would encounter on the unit to which they are assigned for their senior clinical preceptorship. The students are asked to identify what health literacy barriers that specific population of patients might present. At this point in the project, students are not focusing on barriers of an individual patient; instead, they are exploring problems and barriers that might be shared by patients in that specialty population. Thus, students working in maternal-child health have talked about how teachable moments must be seized. Students assigned to the intensive care unit have discussed how they may need to focus on the health literacy needs of a patient's family to help the

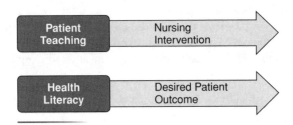

FIGURE 3.1 Outcome-centered health care environment.

family and patient understand the complex nature of the care the patient is receiving. One student assigned to an oncology unit wrote:

> Specifically in oncology, health literacy has yet another barrier: stress. "Cancer" is an extremely scary diagnosis, regardless of how treatable or curable it may be. When physicians speak with patients about their found diagnosis, many patients probably cannot pay attention to any information given after their anxiety-causing diagnosis. Davis et al. (2002) claim "the physician/patient communication literature indicates that immediately after leaving their physicians' offices, patients are able to correctly identify only 50 percent of the critical information just given to them. In these circumstances it is incredibly important to evaluate the level of health literacy of the patient and the information necessary to allow them full access to their care.

Proceeding from this basic foundation, students are then asked to choose an assigned patient and apply what they have learned about culture, language, family dynamics, communication, teaching, learning, motivation, and more. The students are encouraged to synthesize multiple aspects of what they have learned in nursing school and to apply what they know to an individual patient's situation, see the disease through the patient's eyes, then develop interventions to increase the patient's health literacy.

In the following scenario, a student used her knowledge of health literacy to identify barriers and facilitators prior to providing discharge teaching. She identified language and culture as potential barriers to learning, and discovered that important aspects of this patient's care are performed by her son and daughter-in-law. The student then decided to include the family in teaching.

> I met this patient on day two of admission to go over her discharge instructions. I introduced myself and my role and explained that I was there to help her understand her discharge instructions and answer any questions that she may have. Since I speak the patient's native dialect (Punjabi) I was able to communicate with the patient without an interpreter. The patient's husband (also non-English speaking) was sitting by the bedside. I decided that I had to first assess the patient's health literacy deficits before I could do any kind of teaching or information sharing with her. After a short interview where I questioned the patient on her reading and understanding ability, I also found out that the patient's food was prepared by her daughter-in-law and her son filled her 7-day pill dispenser every Sunday. Since the patient's son and daughter-in-law were on their way to the hospital I decided to wait and include them in any further communication. While I waited, I listed the health deficiencies of the patient as follows. There is a language barrier, lack of ability to read and comprehend beyond [about] an 8th-grade level, and unfamiliarity with medical terminology. I was also aware of a cultural barrier—a norm that does not question health care providers—so I knew I had to be gently coaxing to encourage questions.

When students see the disease through the patient's eyes and from the patient's world, new possibilities for interventions emerge. This student speaking in the patient's native language was able to determine that the patient was not the sole source of control and provider of care. The student was able to alter and change teaching by scheduling the teaching time to when other family members who participated in the patient's care were present.

As the student identified, a barrier to improving this patient's health literacy was language. In a multicultural environment this barrier was overcome when the student spoke the same language as the patient; more often, however, the student and patient do not share the same language. Patients with limited English proficiency (LEP) may also have limited health literacy, as was true of the patient in the described scenario; it is recommended that teaching be performed in the patient's primary language or often with the use of interpreters. Attempts to determine if the patient has learned the information being taught are often stymied by specialized vocabulary and cultural nuances. These issues are all considered with this project.

An essential goal for the student to demonstrate that a patient's health literacy is improved is to validate that learning has occurred. Students have accomplished this goal by setting up teach-back situations—having the patient demonstrate a technique or use a simulated model to illustrate a point. In the following scenario, the student and preceptor developed a unique approach to teach the patient how his indwelling urinary catheter works.

A senior male student and his preceptor stepped into a challenging situation at the beginning of their shift. A 60-year-old Asian male who reportedly spoke limited English had just pulled out his indwelling urinary catheter with the balloon intact. The student and nurse entered the room on hearing loud screaming and saw blood covering the bed and patient, and the patient about to pull out his IV. After the student and his preceptor calmed the patient and assisted him to the bathroom then back to bed, the patient continued to bleed. The preceptor and student obtained an order for the catheter to be reinserted. The student related the following sequence of events that ensued:

> [The patient] was beginning to bleed more than a little. My preceptor explained to him that we needed to put the catheter back in to stop his bleeding. He began to speak good English at this point. He did not want it and it appeared to me that he did not comprehend how the balloon worked, why it was not inflated going into his penis but was inflated in his bladder, and then could be deflated to come out. He kept insisting that the balloon would hurt coming out again. I began talking to him and tried to focus exactly on his source of fear and lack of knowledge. He began to listen to me and I really took my time explaining how everything worked. My preceptor said that I should keep talking to him because he was listening to me. My preceptor had the idea to take a Foley kit and demonstrate how it worked for him. We made a bladder with a Styrofoam cup with a hole in the bottom. I showed [the patient] what the tube looked like, how the balloon worked, how it was inflated in the bladder and how it was deflated when it was time to take it out.

The student then allowed the patient to pull on the inflated balloon that was in place in the Styrofoam cup and the patient was able to see the results of what happened. The catheter was successfully reinserted, and the inflated balloon stemmed the flow of blood. The student and preceptor rejoiced at the successful catheter insertion. An hour later the patient called for the student and stated that he wanted to know the nurse's name and the student's name so that he could thank them in writing. Perseverance, patience, and a determination to help the patient understand resulted in a positive outcome for this patient.

Issues with health literacy are not limited to the time of discharge. To promote the safety and comfort of the patient, the preceptor and student demonstrated teamwork in their creative problem solving. This story was reported in the student's final health literacy paper and demonstrates how this individual patient's needs were met. It illustrated the successful performance of multiple QSEN competencies in the areas of patient-centered care, cultural competence, teamwork, and safety.

In a final example, another student is able to meet many aspects of the informatics of QSEN competency as well as demonstrating patient-centered care and meeting a variety of safety concerns.

> I recognized that the short amount of time that I had to teach the patient would only allow me to teach the essential medications that she had to take and the reasons she should return to the hospital or notify her doctor, so I had to come up with a plan. After getting her to tell me the reasons she should be notifying her physician, I documented in her record that she was able to state the reasons that she would have to call and she was able to recall these with accuracy. Then, I gathered all of the information together that I had originally thought I was going to teach and entered it into the area of her EMR [electronic medical record] that shows the teaching plan. This allowed me to focus on the medications, and in the final time before her discharge I worked on getting her to show me which medications she would take each morning and what they were for. In the discharge note, I was able to say that she was able to do this with 100% accuracy.

One of the challenges in all health care settings is the limited timeframes available for teaching. Utilizing the medical record and focusing on just a few essential aspects of the patient's discharge, the student was able to improve the patient's understanding of health care.

This project helps the students understand the amount of patient teaching that must be done to achieve an improvement in the patient's health literacy. Basic aspects of patient teaching, such as not teaching everything to the patient at one time and using return demonstrations and teach backs to demonstrate improved health literacy, are reinforced.

CONCLUSION

The health literacy project described allows students to synthesize what they have learned and integrate it into performance as they teach patients and document that learning has occurred. The health literacy project is one method for students to learn how to improve patient outcomes. It is perhaps best described by one of the students:

> By performing this study I have learned valuable information about ways to teach others. I now know how to use less technical terms and to use handouts. I now realize the effectiveness of return demonstrations in evaluation, and feel that I am able to teach better in the future. Through examination [of health literacy] I feel that I have a more comprehensive knowledge about the barriers to learning and literacy, and also the ways to overcome these issues. I will take this model into consideration when interacting with a patient, and utilize health literacy concepts to evaluate the patient's understanding. If all providers learn to assess their patient's literacy needs, outcomes for all patients can be improved.

References

Cormier, C. M., & Kotrlik, J. W. (2009). Health literacy knowledge and experiences of senior baccalaureate nursing students. *Journal of Nursing Education, 48*(5), 237–248.

Davis, T. C., Williams, M. V., Marin, E., Parker, R. M., & Glass, J. (2002). Health literacy and cancer communication. *CA: A Cancer Journal for Clinicians, 52*, 134–149.

National Patient Safety Foundation (NPSF). (2010). Health literacy statistics. Retrieved from www.npsf.org

Quality and Safety Education for Nurses. (2010). From www.qsen.org

Sudore, R. L., Landefeld, C. S., Perez-Stable, E. J., Bibbins-Domingo, K., Williams, B. A., & Schillinger, D. (2009). Unraveling the relationship between literacy, language proficiency, and patient-physician communication. *Patient Education and Counseling, 25*, 398–402.

Sudore, R. L., Mehta, K. M., Simonsick, E. M., Harris, T. B., Newman, A. B., Satterfield, S., et al. (2006). Limited literacy in older people and disparities in health and healthcare access. *Journal of the American Geriatrics Society, 54*, 770–776.

Sudore, R. L., Yaffe, K., Satterfield, S., Harris, T. B., Mehta, K. M., Simonsick, E. M., et al. (2006). Limited literacy and mortality in the elderly: the health, aging, and body composition study. *Journal of General Internal Medicine, 21*, 806–812.

Trossman, S. (2010). Nurses promote true health understanding through literacy. *American Nurse Today, 5*(9), 32–33.

Educating Meaningful Users: Using the EHR in Nurse Practitioner Education

Mary Jane Cook, MSN, RN, FNP, BC
Katherine J. Dontje, PhD, RN, FNP

Competency in informatics is essential for all health care providers. Knowledge and skill in informatics transforms the health care provider from a data gatherer to a knowledge worker. Nurse practitioner (NP) students, as future providers, must be educated to meet the needs of an increasingly complex technological health care system. Several national nursing organizations have identified the electronic health record (EHR) as an important component of the technology agenda for improving health and quality of patient care. These organizations include the National League for Nursing (NLN, 2008), Quality and Safety Education for Nurses competencies (QSEN, 2011), and the Technology Informatics Guiding Educational Reform (TIGER) Initiative (2010).

The Health Information Technology for Economic and Clinical Health Act (The Office of the National Coordinator for Health Information Technology, 2011) was designed to increase the meaningful use of EHRs in the health care system and to link quality improvement and reimbursement in the clinical setting. Many of the NP informatics competencies and meaningful use criteria can be achieved utilizing the EHR in the education process. Changes in the NP curriculum need to emphasize both knowledge of informatics tools and how to harness these tools to improve quality and safety in patient care. Areas of focus for this quality improvement include clinical decision support tools and reminders designed to improve the utilization of evidence-based guidelines. The EHR also has the potential to enhance quality and safety by influencing prescribing practices of NP students through checking for medication interactions and use of medication reconciliation techniques.

Additional impetus for the EHR project described here was provided by our observation of student clinical experiences. Students are not always allowed access to documents in the EHR at their clinical sites due to security issues. This is particularly true of practices just initiating an EHR system and of small practices. Despite the increasing use of EHRs, NP student access is still limited. NP students need to understand not only how to document, but more importantly, how to use the data for quality and safety purposes. By providing a training experience, we can ensure that all the students in the program have an opportunity to meet the minimum competencies related to the EHR.

EHR PROJECT DESIGN AND IMPLEMENTATION

The NP faculty at Michigan State University (MSU) sought to incorporate informatics into the curriculum to meet the increased emphasis on informatics competencies and the expansion of the EHR in clinical practice. To assist in this curriculum process, faculty applied to the Health Information Technology Scholars (HITS) Program ("Advancing Health Information Technologies, N.D). The HITS program assists faculty in the design and implementation of projects that incorporate health information technology (HIT) into the curriculum. The project planned by faculty at MSU involved mapping the informatics competencies to the course objectives and developing educational activities for NP students to gain knowledge of informatics while improving their EHR skills.

The EHR project was initiated as a collaboration among the NP faculty, medical faculty, and HIT team. The university outpatient clinics use an EHR that can be accessed remotely by providers. A student version of the EHR, financed through a grant from the Health Resources and Services Administration (HRSA), was developed by the medical faculty. The NP program was allocated a portion of the student EHR for use in this project. The modifications made by HIT and access licenses were financed through nursing instructional technology funds.

Informatics competencies, based on the work of Curran (2003), were mapped to the NP clinical courses and accompanied by learning objectives, content, instructional strategies, and evaluation assignments created for each (Box 4.1). The EHR was modified to allow the students to access the record remotely from their home computers throughout

BOX 4.1 EXAMPLE OF ELECTRONIC HEALTH RECORD (EHR) CURRICULUM PLANNING

Competencies Unit Objectives
1. Uses decision support systems, expert systems, and aids for differential diagnosis. Student will demonstrate understanding of guideline integration into the EHR through decision support by completing a patient documentation using a decision support tool.

Unit Content
1. Use of EHR with Framingham cardiovascular risk tool, PHQ-9 depression screening

Instructional Strategies Explanation/Demonstration/Practice
1. EHR Tools (content 1–3)
   a. Demonstrate use of EHR tools (categories of tools)
      i. Disease risk (Framingham cardiovascular risk)
      ii. Diagnostic tools (PHQ-9 depression screening)
   b. Student will record a patient using a tool.

Learner Evaluation Strategies
1. Documentation of a patient forwarded to faculty desktop demonstrating the correct use of a decision support tool

the state. The NP students complete the EHR assignments as part of their course work in a hybrid NP program.

Currently, two cohorts of master-level NP students (2010 and 2011) have used the EHR as part of course assignments. An indication of the surge in outpatient EHR use was demonstrated by NP student reports of experience with an EHR in their NP clinical experiences (19% of Cohort 1 [N = 35] and, 51% of Cohort 2 [N = 42]). This reinforces the imperative to educate NP students as informatics knowledge workers.

PROJECT EVALUATION

Outcomes measured for the project were student satisfaction and knowledge. After each EHR assignment, students were asked to complete a faculty-constructed satisfaction survey (Table 4.1). Students were asked open-ended questions about problems encountered. Knowledge was assessed with a pretest and posttest and by the quality of the student's work on EHR assignments. The largest knowledge gain was in the areas related to the assignment using the EHR. Student EHR assignments were structured with the focus on assessment, health promotion, and outcomes. The assignments consisted of a cardiovascular risk assessment using EHR tools, use of guideline reminders for health screenings and immunizations, and use of the EHR to gather information related to chronic disease outcomes.

TABLE 4.1

Percentage of Students with Agree or Strongly Agree Reaction

Reaction Question	Cohort 1 (N = 30)	Cohort 2 (N = 39)
1. The tutorials helped me access and use the electronic health record (EHR).	28.5%	83.4%
2. The simulated EHR was easy to access.	28.5%	42.9%
3. I learned something new about the electronic health record from this assignment.	78.6%	82.1%
4. The Citrix program was easy to download.	34.5%	60%
5. I was able to log into the simulated EHR without any difficulty.	20.6%	79.5%
6. I am confident that I can access the simulated EHR from home.	57.1%	92.3%
7. I was able to get help accessing the simulated EHR when I needed it.	44.8%	83.3%
8. Using the simulated EHR will make it easier to use other EHRs in my clinical sites.	51.7%	56.4%

Initial remote access to the EHR for Cohort 1 was accomplished by 63.3% of the NP students. Browser security was an initial problem in Cohort 1. An unintended barrier to access occurred for Cohort 1 due to a major upgrade of the EHR system during the time of the assignment. As a result, scrambled letters and numbers appeared on the screen rather than the usual text. The most common student problem was downloading the access software. Students experienced computer shutdown or were unable to complete the installation process. Security for the EHR required two login points. Consequently, forgetting usernames and/or passwords was a common problem. Understandably, students were dissatisfied with the assignment.

The results of the initial EHR assignment pointed to areas for improvement. Remote access to the EHR was clearly a problem for Cohort 1. Lessons learned from our experiences with Cohort 1 helped improve the EHR access for Cohort 2. Several changes were made in the instructions for EHR use. Faculty created instructional videos and screen shots that provided verbal and visual instructions for students. Students were also instructed to bring their computers to campus to walk through downloading the software needed for access. Four computers in the nursing computer lab were designated for use as an alternative access point for EHR assignments. Cohort 2 reaction scores for satisfaction related to access. The confidence level of Cohort 2 improved over Cohort 1. All Cohort 2 students were able to access the EHR remotely.

The lecture on and demonstration of the EHR delivered to Cohort 1 resulted in only a small increase in knowledge from pretest to posttest. In addition to lecture, Cohort 2 was required to complete a risk assessment assignment using the EHR tools. Cohort 2 had a much greater increase in scores on the risk assessment question from pretest to posttest. This difference implies improved knowledge through active learning with the EHR tools.

Incidental observations also informed the EHR project. Faculty were required to function as technology support for the students. It was not unusual for faculty and the information technology team to receive multiple emails daily related to technical problems with the EHR. The information technology team had responsibility only for the software required for access and was available Monday through Friday during regular business hours. Weekend and after hours support was the responsibility of the faculty. A faculty champion in collaboration with a designated support person in HIT was the most efficient means to work through difficulties. Flexibility was essential to improve the experience for the students.

Despite the access problems for Cohort 1, faculty noted that many students chose to include the EHR in their quality improvement papers for their final clinical course. The paper requires students to collaborate with their preceptors to design and plan a quality improvement intervention relevant to the practice site. Data collection of chronic disease metrics, risk assessment, and data reporting to third-party payers are examples of EHR content in the projects. This incidental observation demonstrates the increased awareness of the uses of the EHR for quality improvement and reimbursement.

LESSONS LEARNED

The major goal of this project was to provide online remote access for students to an EHR activity. This was possible through the use of a relatively low-cost version of the EHR employed in the university's outpatient clinics. Faculty planning similar projects should be aware of implications for faculty and student assignments. Considerations include the time spent in choosing and developing an EHR system and understanding the strengths and limitations of the system, as well as possible barriers to student and faculty access. In addition, a great deal of faculty time is needed to facilitate student access to the EHR system.

The key concept to consider when developing new experiences in the curriculum is that the technology should facilitate, not inhibit, student learning. Students should learn the practical application of EHR use and data rather than the technical aspects of the software and data entry.

Additional attention should be paid to the cost of using an EHR system and how this can be built into the budget. Depending on the system chosen, cost and usability can vary widely. At our university, we were able to take advantage of a system developed through an HRSA grant by the medical faculty. The cost was minimal because of the work completed prior to the implementation of the EHR in the NP curriculum. Expenses included payment for programming and for site licenses. To control costs, we limited the site licenses to six and assigned students times when they could use the system. Licensing costs are ongoing, requiring collaboration with our instructional technology department to budget for continued use of the system by students.

CONCLUSION

To prepare NP students for practice, it has become increasingly important for schools of nursing to address how technology and, in particular, EHRs, can impact the quality and reimbursement of their practice. It is essential that the curriculum address quality, safety, and reimbursement issues to prepare students with the skills to appropriately interact with the technology to meet national initiatives. By providing students with the skills and knowledge to use the EHR as a tool for quality improvement, they will be better prepared as active members of the health care team.

Research should be ongoing to discover how the use of an EHR system influences students' learning and their ability to meet the NP informatics competencies. This is especially true with the emergence of the DNP Essentials (American Association of Colleges of Nursing [AACN], 2006) and NP competencies (National Organization of Nurse Practitioner Faculties [NONPF], 2012) incorporating the expanded expectations of technology knowledge and skills. Future research studies could evaluate EHR systems and which are most effective for student learning. In addition, research regarding how to integrate EHR activities into NP clinical experiences to improve care quality and scholarship can inform future curriculum changes.

References

Advancing Health Information Technologies through Faculty Empowerment. (N.D.). Health Information Technology Scholars Program. Retrieved from http://www.hits-colab.org/

American Association of Colleges of Nursing (AACN). (2006). The Essentials of Doctoral Education for Advanced Nursing Practice. Retrieved from www.aacn.nche.edu/publications/position/DNPEssentials.pdf

Curran, C. R. (2003). Informatics competencies for nurse practitioners. *AACN Clinical Issues, 14*(3), 320–330. doi: 10.1097/00044067-200308000-00007

National League for Nursing (NLN) (2008). Preparing the next generation of nurses to practice in a technology-rich environment: An informatics agenda. Retrieved from www.nln.org/aboutnln/PositionStatements/informatics_052808.pdf

National Organization of Nurse Practitioner Faculties (NONPF). (2012). Nurse practitioner core competencies. Retrieved from www.nonpf.com/associations/10789/files/NPCoreCompetenciesFinal2012.pdf

Quality and Safety Education for Nurses (QSEN). (2011). Competency Knowledge, Skills, and Attitudes (Graduate): Informatics. Retrieved from www.qsen.org/ksas_graduate.php#informatics

The Office of the National Coordinator for Health Information Technology. (2011). Electronic Health Records and Meaningful Use. Retrieved from http://healthit.hhs.gov/portal/server.pt?open=512&objID=2996&mode=2.

The Technology Informatics Guiding Educational Reform Initiative. (2010). Informatics competencies for every practicing nurse: Recommendations from the TIGER Collaborative. Retrieved from www.tigersummit.com/Competencies_New_B949.html

5

Integration of Informatics Concepts and Applications throughout a BSN to DNP Curriculum

Vicki J. Brownrigg, PhD, RN, FNP-C
Mary Enzman-Hines, PhD, APRN, CNS, CPNP, APHN-BC

Health information technology (HIT) is projected to play a vital role in transforming health care delivery in the United States by improving the quality and efficiency of health care systems (Marcotte et al., 2012). However, the Institute of Medicine Committee on Patient Safety and Health Information Technology (IOM, 2011) concluded this transformation can take place only when HIT is appropriately designed and implemented. The American Association of Colleges of Nursing (AACN, 2006, 2011) now includes requirements for the inclusion of health care technology content as part of the essential core competencies that are to be acquired over the course of graduate nursing students' educational programs. Additionally, the position statement of the National League for Nursing (NLN) on technology and informatics in nursing education provides recommendations for the integration of HIT learning activities and outcomes at all academic levels of nursing education (NLN, 2008). It is within the NLN recommendations that this project was first envisioned by two graduate nursing faculty members.

This Health Information Technology Scholars (HITS) project sought to integrate health informatics didactic and experiential learning throughout a newly established online BSN to DNP curriculum. Specific aims for the project were to:

1. Integrate informatics into every course in the BSN to DNP curriculum

2. Develop faculty skills in the delivery of informatics content in the BSN to DNP online curriculum

3. Prepare all DNP graduates with the knowledge and skills necessary to seamlessly utilize a broad array of informatics applications in advanced practice nursing (APN)

PROJECT DEVELOPMENT

This project began with the selection of two faculty members into the HITS program. The HITS program is supported by a Health Resources and Service Administration (HRSA) five-year grant awarded to a collaboration of four schools of nursing in partnership with the NLN. The program was designed to "develop, implement, disseminate, and sustain a faculty development collaborative (FDC) initiative to integrate information technologies in nursing curricula and expand the capacity of collegiate schools of nursing to educate students for the 21st century" (NLN, n.d., paragraph 2).

During the project's initial phase, the decision was made to integrate nursing informatics concepts, applications, and practice throughout the curriculum, as opposed to offering a single informatics course. The emerging development of the courses within the new curriculum supported the idea that integration would provide students the opportunity to progressively and seamlessly assimilate informatics into their role as APNs by applying informatics concepts and practices throughout their DNP coursework.

The integration of the informatics content throughout the curriculum was based on the work of the Technology Informatics Guiding Education Reform (TIGER) competencies collaborative. The TIGER competencies are placed within three major categories:

1. Basic computer competencies

2. Information literacy

3. Information management (TIGER, 2009)

Additionally, the AACN Essentials (2006), National Organization of Nurse Practitioner Faculty competencies (NONPF, 2006), and NP informatics competencies (Curran, 2003) were compared for overlap as well as unique characteristics, and placed within one of the three components of the TIGER competency model. A list of HIT topics and skills structured within the TIGER competencies and integrated throughout the curriculum is shown in Box 5.1.

Curriculum Development and Implementation

Basic Computer Competencies

As a result of the HITS project, basic computer competencies were integrated throughout all courses in the new curriculum. Computer competencies applied throughout the curriculum include:

- E-learning in a fully online environment
- Email communication
- Recorded presentations using commercial presentation software
- Utilization of word processing for scholarly papers and online course discussions

The development and use of databases and spreadsheets are required in statistics and organizational systems/leadership courses as well as the final capstone projects when

BOX 5.1 KEY HIT AND INFORMATICS SKILLS

Basic Computer Competencies
E-learning–online curriculum
Word processing and scholarly papers using American Psychological Association (APA) format
Online PowerPoint presentations
Email communication
Recorded online webinar presentations
Online video communications
Wiki/blog development
Development/use of databases and spreadsheets
SPSS database development and statistical analysis

Information Literacy
Online search engines
University library Ovid searches
Scholarly papers requiring APA reference list and citations

Information Management
Electronic health records (EHR) selection and use
Personal health records (PHR)
Clinical decision support (CDS)
Electronic prescribing
Computerized provider order entry (CPOE)
Auto ID/barcoding
Standardized terminology
Health information exchanges
Integration and interoperability
Data entry, aggregation, extraction, and analysis for quality improvement
Data entry, aggregation, extraction, and analysis for financial management
Evidence-based practice project requiring outcomes evaluation
Informatics applications appropriate for entrepreneurial project
Policy/law (Accountable Care Act, HITECH, HIPAA, EHR requirement, meaningful use, certification)
Privacy
Security
Ethics
Telehealth

appropriate. Additionally, synchronous, online video communications, recorded webinar presentations, wikis, and blogs are used to facilitate social learning in select courses.

Information Literacy

The TIGER competencies (2009) define *information literacy* as "the ability to identify information needed for a specific purpose, locate pertinent information, evaluate the information, and apply it correctly" (p. 5). All courses throughout the BSN to DNP curriculum emphasize the application of information literacy by requiring the use of university library Ovid and online search engines for the development of all scholarly papers. Proper citation of references is required in all online group discussions. Throughout the curriculum, faculty members emphasize the use of reputable reference sources and assist students in identifying those online sites that are appropriate for scholarly papers, patient teaching, and delivery of patient care. Supplemental written and audiovisual tutorials on information literacy are provided to students as they enter the DNP program by the university librarian assigned to the College of Nursing. These tutorials are imbedded in every BSN to DNP online course.

Information Management

Information management is defined by TIGER (2009) as "a process consisting of 1) collecting data, 2) processing the data, and 3) presenting and communicating the processed data as information or knowledge" (p. 7). Concepts and specific applications of information management are initially introduced in the first semester to students in the organizational systems/leadership course. This includes an overview of electronic health records (EHRs) for the management and analysis of data for evaluation of patient outcomes, evidence-based practice, and quality improvement. Other HIT concepts and skills introduced in this course and subsequently applied in later courses include (a) standardized terminology; (b) integration and interoperability of HIT systems; and (c) privacy, and security related to HIT.

The business, finance, and entrepreneurship course requires students to select appropriate HIT applications for an entrepreneurial project. This course also emphasizes the entry, aggregation, extraction, and analysis of data for financial management.

In the advanced health care policy, law, and ethics course, students discuss HIT policy and law including the Health Information Technology for Economic and Clinical Health Act (HITECH); Health Insurance Portability and Accountability Act (HIPAA), privacy, and security related to HIT; implementation and meaningful use of EHRs by 2014; EHR certification; and ethics related to HIT. The role of HIT in evidence-based practice and translational research is explored in the evidence-based practice course before students develop their capstone project proposals. Finally, information management skills and competencies are integrated throughout the students' clinical and practicum experiences. These include hands-on use of electronic and personal health records, clinical decision support, electronic prescribing, computerized provider order entry, and auto ID/barcoding.

Faculty Development

Similar to survey findings cited by the NLN (2008), little knowledge and understanding of HIT and health care informatics existed among the nursing faculty; therefore, faculty development was a critical consideration in integrating informatics throughout the curriculum. A two-step approach was taken to assist faculty in the process of integration. First, one-on-one faculty consultation was provided to facilitate the inclusion of appropriate informatics content and learning activities in each course. Additionally, a workshop on e-learning was provided. Additional HIT and e-learning presentations for the faculty are currently in the planning stages.

RESULTS

Each course in the new curriculum with the integrated informatics content has been delivered at least one time. Students no longer report a sense of dread upon hearing the term "informatics" and often articulate how the addition of information technology can improve safety and quality in their APN practices when implemented appropriately. Additionally, DNP students are increasingly selecting HIT topics for their clinical practicum and capstone projects. The long-term project outcome to prepare DNP graduates with the knowledge and skills necessary to seamlessly utilize a broad array of informatics applications in APN will be formally evaluated using graduate and employer surveys six months after student completion of the BSN to DNP curriculum. This formal evaluation had not yet occurred because there had not been graduates from the new BSN to DNP curriculum at the time of this writing.

This project is in its infancy and, like all curriculum development, will likely never be fully complete. Health care technology is developing faster than it can be adequately implemented; thus, inclusion of informatics in nursing education curricula will require constant revision. A major lesson learned during the implementation of this HITS project is that it is imperative for nurse educators, practitioners, and students to continually expand their knowledge and skills in HIT and nursing informatics as they progress through the second decade of the 21st century and beyond.

References

American Association of Colleges of Nursing (AACN). (2006). The essentials of doctoral education for advanced nursing practice. Retrieved from www.aacn.nche.edu/dnp.

American Association of Colleges of Nursing (AACN). (2011). The Essentials of Master's Education in Nursing. Retrieved from http://www.aacn.nche.edu/education-resources/essential-series.

Curran, C. (2003). Informatics competencies for nurse practitioners. *AACN Clinical Issues: Advanced Practice In Acute & Critical Care, 14*(3), 320–330.

Institute of Medicine Committee on Patient Safety and Health Information Technology (2011). *Health IT and Patient Safety: Building Safer Systems for Better Care.* Retrieved from www.nap.edu/catalog.php?record_id=13269.

Marcotte, L., Seidman, J., Trudel, K., Berwick, D. M., Blumenthal, D., Mostashari, F., & Jain, S. H. (2012). Achieving meaningful use of health information technology. *Archives of Internal Medicine, 172*(9), 731–736.

National League for Nursing (NLN). (2008). Preparing the next generation of nurses to practice in a technology-rich environment: An informatics agenda. Retrieved from www.nln.org/aboutnln/PositionStatements/index.htm.

National League of Nursing (NLN). (n.d.). HITS website. Retrieved from http://www.hits-colab.org/

National Organization of Nurse Practitioner Faculty (NONPF). (2006). Practice doctorate nurse practitioner entry-level competencies. Retrieved from www.nonpf.com/display-common.cfm?an=1&subarticlenbr=14.

Technology Informatics Guiding Educational Reform (TIGER). (2009). TIGER Informatics Competencies Collaborative (TICC) Final Report. Retrieved from www.thetigerinitiative.org/resources.aspx.

Putting It All Together:
A Multidisciplinary, Multi-Institutional Clinical Simulation Center

Carolyn B. Yucha, PhD, RN, FAAN

Shirlee J. Snyder, EdD, RN

Miriam E. Bar-on, MD, FAAP

David Frommer, AIA, NCARB

Lance Baily, BA, EMT

The Clinical Simulation Center of Las Vegas (CSCLV) opened in August, 2009. This 31,000-square foot area was designed to meet the annual simulation and skills training requirements for more than 650 BSN nursing students, medical students, and medical and surgical residents from three different universities located within the same geographic area. Upon completion of the CSCLV, a series of interprofessional cases were developed for the nursing and medical students from the universities involved in the project to provide simulation educational experiences in teamwork and collaboration of health care professionals.

BACKGROUND

In the fall of 2006, the deans of nursing at the University of Nevada Las Vegas and at Nevada State College discussed the simulation resources needed for their schools. At that time, each school owned a high-fidelity human patient simulator, but neither had the faculty, technicians, and funds to effectively incorporate this technology into its educational programs. As a potential solution, the deans recommended a collaborative simulation center be developed. Due to the immense number of factors related to the creation of this center, this undertaking was far more complicated than anticipated.

This project aligned with the vision of the chancellor of the Nevada System of Higher Education (NSHE), who desired the creation of a unified health sciences system that would encourage collaboration between public colleges and universities in the area. With the chancellor's support, the proposed simulation center was allocated $15.75 million in state Capital Improvement Program funds by the legislature in the spring of 2007, with the funds designated for the center's design, construction, and equipment. By the summer of 2007, the University of Nevada School of Medicine (UNSOM) joined the venture, and the task of designing this interprofessional, multi-institutional educational facility began.

To satisfy the center's unique goals, the group analyzed other collaborative health-related programs:

- Fellowship programs in pediatric critical care medicine (Nishisaki, Hales, Biagas, et al., 2009) developed a "boot-camp" for fellows' orientation using the combined resources of institutions in a defined geographic region to attain better training.
- In Oregon, a statewide implementation of simulation training also capitalized on the concept of collaborating across institutions for a common goal (Seropian, Dillman, & Farris, 2007).
- Multiple sources have advocated multidisciplinary or interprofessional education (Barnsteiner, Disch, Hall, Mayer, & Moore, 2007; IOM, 1999) as a critical method to deliver training to future health professionals, and studies evaluating the presentation of experiential, interprofessional education through simulation for nursing and medical students have demonstrated better communication and improved patient care (Dillon, Noble, & Kaplan, 2009; Reese, Jeffries, & Engum, 2010).

Despite these successful examples, no similar process had been attempted in Nevada. Although an interinstitutional, interprofessional collaboration would enable each school to implement educational opportunities for its learners that would not be feasible if attempted independently, the task of developing and operating such a center was complex. To enable others to learn from the CSCLV process, in this article we:

- Describe the funding sources of the CSCLV
- Describe the space planning process to build the CSCLV
- Describe the administrative commitments necessary
- Describe the process used to develop the staffing requirements and to hire and orient new staff
- Provide lessons learned

FUNDING

Space for the CSCLV was available in a building recently purchased and earmarked for collaborative learning, but the specific usage plan had not yet been developed. The 2007 state legislature allocated $15.75 million for the design, extensive remodeling, and fixed furnishings (e.g., cabinetry, plumbing, lighting) for the 31,000-square foot space. The three participating institutions developed a memorandum of understanding (MOU) to cover operations and management costs not funded by the state, including electricity, maintenance, security, and other necessary continuous services, and a contribution to debt service relative to campus improvements. The development of the MOU and charges to the respective institutions were based on each institution's estimated number of students and square foot usage. Consequently, the two nursing schools involved in the project cover 80 percent of the expenses (i.e., a 40-40-20 split among the three institutions).

Additional funding sources were needed for the following expenses: B-Line® integrative software, computers, televideo and audiovisual equipment, document cameras, high-fidelity simulators, ultrasound machine, MedEx™ medication delivery systems, and additional task trainers. Fortunately, two federal earmarks, totaling $2 million, supplemented state funding for the purchase of these items.

To cover the costs for operating the center, including staffing, supplies, software, and equipment maintenance, an increase in student fees was warranted. These fees, again using the 40-40-20 ratio, were derived from estimated costs of the operations budget and the anticipated number of students. In the nursing programs, the fees were attached to four or five courses at $300 per course; in the medical school, they were established as $577 annual program fees for each student during the final two years of medical school. Usage statistics are being kept to analyze the initial funding distribution with an eye toward modification when needed.

Students were informed of the additional fees and a proposal was sent to the NSHE Board of Regents. The request was approved in the spring of 2009 and took effect the following fall. Although student fee increases are generally not approved, these were approved, as the Board of Regents agreed that this collaborative program provided an excellent opportunity to integrate simulation into both nursing and medical school curricula.

Because the funds from the newly established fees were unavailable until the fall of 2009, the NSHE executive vice chancellor contributed an additional $92,000 to hire and orient three technical staff and for necessary preparations for the CSCLV's opening in late August 2009. As student fees could not be used for administrative positions, including a director and an administrative assistant, two of the schools contributed funds for these additional positions. Each institution contributed its available equipment to ensure resources were in place when classes began.

Table 6.1 shows the six initial funding sources for the CSCLV. Obtaining additional funding sources by proposing collaborative ventures is more efficient than attempting to obtain funds as an individual university. Therefore, plans for future funding are

TABLE 6.1

Initial Sources of Funding for CSCLV

Funding Source	Amount	Primary Use
State legislature	$15.75 million	Construction
Federal appropriation	$2 million	Equipment and software
Student fees	$365,000 annually	Support staff and supplies
NSHE health sciences	$92,000	Interim funding for staff; other operating costs
Institutions	$150,000 annually	Director and administrative support
Institutions	In-kind	Equipment and supplies

focused on expanding the collaborative efforts among the current partners, as well as on providing and supporting educational programs for external groups using the capabilities of the CSCLV.

SPACE PLANNING PROCESS

Prior to this project, the health sciences faculty and staff at the three institutions had not worked closely together. To plan the center, however, developing relationships was imperative. Representatives from each educational entity began meeting, initially weekly, to discuss the needs of their learners, including space and time requirements.

Following this initial step, facility design meetings were held. In 2007 and 2008, architects and engineers had removed all nonsupporting walls and materials from a former rehabilitation center that had contained a swimming pool and racquetball courts. The architects were assisted in their work, especially in the consideration of technical and space planning issues, by the UNLV Planning and Construction Department and representatives from the three schools.

The final space design plan consisted of eight primary use areas:

1. Two surgical simulation rooms
2. Three clinical skills rooms
3. Four classrooms
4. Five high-fidelity simulation rooms
5. A 12-room standardized patient suite
6. Student study areas and lounge
7. Faculty and staff offices
8. Facility support spaces

The facility support spaces included space for mechanical, electronic data, and telecommunication services; computer servers; custodial storage; and restrooms. Because females represent 90% of the nursing and 50% of the medical profession workforce, extra women's restrooms were included in the planning, necessitating a waiver of standard building requirements regarding restroom gender assignment. The end product, the CSCLV, became a functional and equitable space designed for the three schools' projected outcomes (see Table 6.2).

Once the physical space was designed, the architects worked with other specialists to integrate and finalize the details of the plan, including the purchase of technical equipment. Representatives discussed televideo, audiovisual, and software functionality, purchase, and installation. The final plan was then sent for bid, as required by state regulations. A construction company was selected to deliver the project via a "construction manager at risk" delivery method. This is a method in which the construction company provides consulting services during the design process for construction feasibility, scheduling, and cost estimating and, when the design is complete, provides a guaranteed maximum price to construct the improvements per the design. Construction began in late fall of 2008, and was complete and ready for occupancy for the fall 2009 semester.

TABLE 6.2

CSCLV Space Allocations

Space	Primary Users	Area (sq ft)
2 Clinical skill labs	Nursing	1,200 each
12-bed hospital ward	Nursing	2,000
Standardized patient suite	Medicine	2,250
80-seat lecture hall	All	2,000
3 (25-seat) classrooms	All	700 each
High-fidelity simulation suite	All	3,600
Surgical simulation	Medicine	1,200
Office space	All	1,400
Student study/lounge spaces	All	1,100
General/custodial storage	All	1,200
Building support spaces	All	6,500

ADMINISTRATIVE COMMITMENTS

While the facility was being designed, a subgroup of the planning committee, the Advisory Committee, worked on the operations plan. This committee comprised the deans of both schools of nursing, the associate dean for graduate medical education from the school of medicine, and a representative of the NSHE. It had three main tasks:

1. Ensure that the educational needs of the participating institutions were met, given the CSCLV space and resources
2. Determine how to fund the center's operation
3. Determine and recruit appropriate staff

Meetings were generally held biweekly over the course of 18 months before the center opened. Open discussions during these meetings led to decisions for center operations, hiring, and policy development.

Because the two nursing schools had approximately equal numbers of students, both schools revised the skills portion of their first-semester coursework to be identical and have the same access to the CSCLV resources. The medical school's needs differed from those of the nursing schools, and the medical students and residents (depending on their specific program or rotation) used different aspects of the center, allowing for a symbiotic relationship between the learners from the three institutions. At all times, the needs of the learners were given priority in the decision-making process. Administrative decisions were made with input from all parties, with compromises made when potential conflicts arose.

This administrative group continues to provide oversight for the CSCLV. Space scheduling is based on student and course requirements. Schedules are requested up to six months in advance so that any scheduling conflicts can be resolved. Last-minute requests are accommodated when possible. Because the center was specifically designed to accommodate large numbers of students participating in a variety of learning experiences, competition for space is not as challenging as might be expected. The good working relationships of the deans and faculty also aid the scheduling process.

STAFFING REQUIREMENTS

The Advisory Committee discussed the support staff requirements to meet the educational needs of the CSCLV. Organizational charts were developed, revised, and finalized depending on each school's needs, expectations, and overall funding. Initially, the Advisory Committee determined that minimum staffing should include two simulation technicians, a lab assistant to facilitate skills training and track supplies, and a director to oversee the center. The Advisory Committee members then served as the search committee to fill these positions.

Because the field of health care simulation is rather new, hiring experienced health care simulation technicians was a challenge. Therefore, simulation technicians were selected based on their backgrounds in either health care or technology, work ethic, interpersonal and organizational skills, ability to work as a team, and comfort with ambiguity. Significant "on-the-job training" occurred until proficiency was attained. Funding was provided for technicians to attend simulation-focused professional conferences and training events.

Initially, two simulation technicians and a laboratory assistant were hired several months before the center opened. This allowed time for these new employees to be oriented to the NSHE, its associated policies and procedures, and their new roles. These new staff members were provided offices at one institution and spent their orientation time becoming familiar with the schools' curricula, learning to manage the simulators, developing familiarity with the equipment, mastering clinical skills, and meeting with faculty and staff of all three institutions.

It became obvious to the Advisory Committee that the center needed a director. One of the initial simulation technicians was hired as the director. In reassessing the position description of the simulation technician and reviewing the technical equipment in the center (including approximately 125 computers), it was determined that the simulation technician position needed to change to accommodate the need for onsite information technology (IT) expertise. The position description was revised and posted, and a technician to provide IT support as well as simulation support was hired. Thus, position descriptions were adjusted even before the CSCLV opened.

Because additional funding was available, an administrative assistant position was created. The administrative assistant role is to purchase supplies, track income/expenses, and organize scheduling. With the exception of the director and administrative assistant positions, student fees fund the staff positions. The current organizational chart is shown in Figure 6.1.

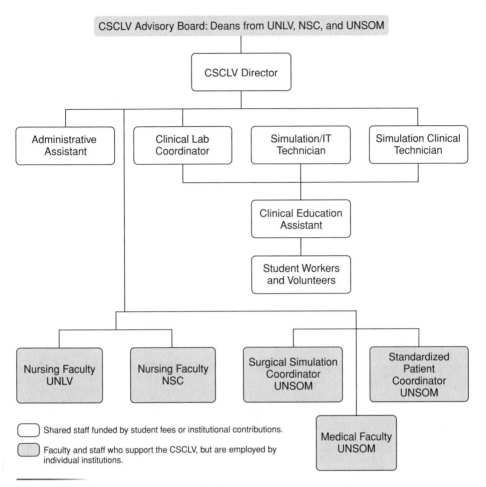

FIGURE 6.1 CSCLV organizational chart.

LESSONS LEARNED

Although the creation of the CSCLV took significant resources, time, and investments, the outcomes meet the needs of all the collaborating institutions by providing their respective learners the opportunity to be educated in a state-of-the-art facility. For institutions that desire to create a collaborative, interinstitutional, interprofessional simulation center similar to the CSCLV, the following points should be considered:

- Plan to invest far more time in collaborative projects than individual ones. The outcomes from collaboration are much greater than the sum of the parts.
- Identify the stakeholders early in the process. Ensure that each has well-defined goals and objectives as well as the authority to make decisions.
- To create a successful collaboration, take time to develop relationships and build trust among participants. Expect chaos and ambiguity, and be

prepared to adapt behaviors as well as revise policies and procedures as new issues arise. All institutional representatives must recognize the need for, and be willing to agree to, compromises that result in a win-win for everyone involved.

- Take advantage of participants' knowledge and skills. Although there does not have to be a clear leader, everyone must contribute to the group based on his or her areas of expertise.

- Take time to reflect on achievements when it seems as though progress is not forthcoming.

CONCLUSIONS

Building the CSCLV was a tremendous undertaking, but the completed facility meets and exceeds the expectations of its users. Serving the needs of nursing and medical students and medical residents, the CSCLV is an example of the benefits that develop when collaborations among educational institutions take place. Collaborative training in simulation methodology has been implemented, and integrated institutional committees created to establish directions for the center. A series of interprofessional cases has been developed as a result of the collaborative training. Interprofessional learning experiences are being developed for the center's users and are gradually being implemented.

The CSCLV places our state at the forefront of nursing and medical innovation and stands as a model for interprofessional educational opportunities. It will continue to do so for years to come.

References

Barnsteiner, J. H., Disch, J. M., Hall, L., Mayer, D., & Moore, S. M. (2007). Promoting interprofessional education. *Nursing Outlook, 55*(3), 144–150.

Dillon, P. M., Noble, K. A., & Kaplan, L. (2009). Simulation as a means to foster collaborative interdisciplinary education. *Nursing Education Perspectives, 30*(2), 87–90.

Institute of Medicine (IOM). (1999). *To err is human: building a safer health system.* Washington, DC: National Academies of Science.

Nishisaki, A., Hales, R., Biagas, K., Cheifetz, I., Corriveau, C., & Nadkarni, V. (2009).

A multi-institutional high fidelity simulation "boot camp" orientation and training program for first year pediatric critical care fellows. *Pediatric Critical Care Medicine, 10,* 157–162.

Reese, C. E., Jeffries, P. R., & Engum, S. A. (2010). Using simulations to develop nursing and medical student collaboration. *Nursing Education Perspectives, 31*(1), 33–37.

Seropian, M., Dillman, D., & Farris, D. (2007). Statewide simulation systems: the next step for anesthesiology. *Anesthesiology Clinics, 25,* 271–282.

7

Establishing the Role of a Quality and Safety Officer in a School of Nursing

Elizabeth Ellen Cooper, DNP, RN, CNE, CNL

For more than a decade, health care providers have talked about ways to provide safe patient care. In 1999, the Institute of Medicine (IOM) published a landmark report, *To Err is Human: Building a Safer Health System,* that was the genesis of this discussion. The report noted that 44,000 to 98,000 patient deaths occur yearly because of errors (IOM, 1999). A 2001 follow-up report, *Crossing the Quality Chasm: A New Health System for the 21st Century,* documented the large gap between what could exist in health care and what actually does exist for all patients (IOM, 2001). Increasing transparency in all areas of health care is one proposed change that may increase patient safety (Cooper, 2012; Kurtzman & Jennings, 2008).

Transparency in reporting errors is a huge challenge in the health care environment (Karlsen, Hendrix, & O'Malley, 2009). *Transparency,* in this case, means that all information regarding medical errors and near misses is disclosed. The key concept in transparency is that all people in a medical organization feel free to report errors and near-miss events. The Institute of Medicine (1999) defined *error* as "failure of a planned action to be completed as intended or the use of a wrong plan to achieve an aim" (p. 28). Near-miss events are "almost" moments, when the almost error is caught before it reaches the patient, and cannot harm the patient (Kessels-Habraken, Van der Schaaf, De Jonge, & Rutte, 2010). With increased reporting, we could evaluate the actual problems and correct the situations that led to errors. In an ideal world, transparency would be a common practice in our health care institutions. However, multiple challenges and barriers to medical reporting exist: dysfunctional reporting systems, fear of liability, lack of time, personal guilt, and blame are just a few of the factors that build barriers to transparency (Madden & Milligan, 2004; Paterick, Paterick, Waterhouse & Paterick, 2009).

Nurses play a significant role in providing safe patient care. Due to the large amount of time they spend at the bedside, they make major contributions in identifying errors and near-miss events (Hession-Laband & Mantell, 2011). Although nurses provide direct patient care error and near-miss reports more often than physicians, the reporting pattern is still in need of improvement and consistency (Rowin et al., 2008).

The literature on medical errors and near-miss reporting primarily discusses the role of physicians and nurses in hospital settings (Flynn, Liang, Dickson, Xie, & Suh, 2012; Hession-Laband & Mantell, 2011; Paterick, Z., Paterick, B., Waterhouse & Paterick, T., 2009). But where does the student nurse stand? When using the key words *student nurse, error reporting,* and *transparency,* no literature is found. A big gap is seen in the literature about transparency related to error and near-miss reporting among student nurses. Student nurses need to be included in reporting to increase both transparency and safe patient care. Student nurses must graduate with all the skills and knowledge needed to provide safe patient care and to bring that knowledge forward the moment they walk into a health care institution as newly licensed registered nurses (Sherwood, 2010). Although nursing schools are responsible for teaching patient safety, teaching to report errors and near misses is what is inconsistently addressed and even missing in many nursing curricula (Howard, 2010).

Identifying and reporting error and near-miss events should be equally important to health care institutions and schools of nursing (Pauly-O'Neill, 2009). Historically, student nurses follow the policy of the health care institution where they are completing their clinical rotation. Working alongside a nurse, the student follows the advice of that particular nurse. If a student is working with a nurse who does not identify or report errors, will the student follow that pattern? Will the identification and incident report be completed?

Student nurses must also report errors and near-miss events to their instructors. The instructors should facilitate following the institution's policies of communicating with the physician, nurse manager, and patient, as well as filing incident report documentation. If the nursing school has further instructions provided in the course syllabus, those should be completed as well.

Often, school of nursing faculty do not report errors and near-miss events. This means that events happen in a silo environment (Sherwood, 2010). If transparency increases safety for our patients, should this not include schools of nursing? Who is monitoring reporting and transparency in nursing schools?

Over the past 10 years, the Robert Wood Johnson Foundation has funded an initiative to assist nursing faculty to bring quality and safety components into schools of nursing. Over the past 10 years, the Quality and Safety Education for Nurses (QSEN) team developed multiple competencies that prepare nurses with the necessary knowledge, skills, and attitudes to improve quality and safety for patients. These QSEN competencies include patient-centered care, evidence-based practice, teamwork and collaboration, informatics, quality improvement, and safety (Cronenwett et al., 2007).

To bring safety to the forefront at a school of nursing, someone must take the lead role. Due to interest sparked by the QSEN, the idea of creating a quality and safety officer (QSO) was developed.

CREATION OF A QUALITY AND SAFETY OFFICER ROLE

The role of a QSO was created in an effort to incorporate QSEN competencies into the nursing curriculum. The belief that safety and transparency need to be a priority in schools of nursing was the driving force. Developing a transparent safety culture in schools of nursing is the long-term goal.

Setting Goals

A beginning step in the development of the QSO role was to create clear goals. The main goal was to identify the safety culture at the school of nursing, then create a plan to enhance safety and transparency with error and near-miss reporting as the priority. Ideas to accomplish this included:

- Identify current reporting methods and enhance the reporting culture in the school of nursing by increasing reporting methods, knowledge, and use among students and faculty members.
- Advance reporting and transparency knowledge.
- Decrease the gap in reporting errors and near-miss events.
- Disseminate reporting results among faculty, students, and health care partners.

Designing the Role

The QSO role required a creative, self-motivated, full-time faculty member with a strong interest in safety. Because there are few QSOs in schools of nursing, the role was created without the use of a template. The title of quality and safety officer was selected for this role to bring a familiar title already in use in health care settings into academia.

Seeking Administrative Support

Seeking support from the dean of the school of nursing was an important initial step. The dean was the key player to facilitate introducing and integrating this major change in safety reporting in the school of nursing. The vision of a QSO was clearly outlined to the dean, including the important contributions this position would have for the school of nursing (see Box 7.1). Next, the dean and QSO jointly introduced this new position to the school of nursing faculty.

BOX 7.1 CONTRIBUTIONS OF THE QUALITY AND SAFETY OFFICER

- Acknowledged as a formal position in the school of nursing.
- Serve as a liaison to administration, faculty, and students regarding safety issues.
- Create a safety vision for the school of nursing.
- Develop ongoing methods to enhance safety and transparency in the school of nursing.

BOX 7.2 ASSESSMENT QUESTIONS

- Is safety discussed at faculty meetings?
- Is safety woven throughout the curriculum?
- Is there a formal reporting system for errors and near misses?
- Do faculty know what errors and near misses are occurring in the school of nursing?
- Do students know what errors and near misses are occurring in the school of nursing?
- Is there a safety policy in place?
- Has transparency ever been discussed at the school of nursing?
- Is there a list of examples of transparency in the school of nursing?

Implementing the Role

The first step in implementing the QSO role was to assess safety and error reporting in the school of nursing. Box 7.2 lists the basic questions used in this assessment.

Applying these questions, it became apparent that safety was an important component in the school of nursing, but was not formalized in regular discussions at faculty meetings or formally addressed in course syllabi. Although safety of the patient and safety education were identified as important to the faculty, the school of nursing did not have a formal error reporting system in place, except to follow the health care institution's policy. This meant that consistency in reporting to the nursing faculty or students was not done.

Once the assessment was completed, the QSO developed an error and near-miss reporting procedure with the goal of increasing transparency in the school of nursing. Transparency in this situation means that error and near-miss reporting is shared with faculty and students. The project's goal was to change the reporting culture in the school of nursing from a closed communication system to a transparent system.

A literature search was completed on the topics of safety and near-miss reporting and transparency. A gap was identified between student error and near-miss reports and transparency in the school of nursing. The gap analysis identified the lack of a formal reporting system on errors and near misses to administration, faculty, and the nursing students. Due to this lack of process, often no report was made or shared. This analysis led to the creation of data collection forms that provide a standard procedure for documentation. The reporting forms are located in the clinical syllabi and are accessible electronically. The clinical faculty share the process with their individual clinical groups.

After completion of the reporting forms by the student or faculty member, the reporting forms are returned to the QSO. Then, a summary dashboard and detailed summary are created. When an error occurs, a root cause analysis (RCA) is completed. The RCA allows all parties involved the opportunity to discuss the error event. An error event often has multiple components and it is through an RCA that these components are identified (Lambton & Mahlmeister, 2010). The QSO facilitates the RCA. The student involved in the error, the preceptor, instructor, unit manager, and chair of the department are all

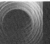

BOX 7.3 QUALITY AND SAFETY OFFICER ACTIVITIES

- Join the curriculum committee.
- Evaluate safety components throughout the curriculum.
- Facilitate incorporating safety education throughout the curriculum.
- Provide safety education updates to faculty and students.
- Disseminate school of nursing reporting information.
- Create a partnership with service.
- Evaluate safety reporting.
- Conduct root cause analysis.
- Evaluate the role of the QSO.
- Disseminate safety information to health care institutions through publications and presentations.

encouraged to attend the RCA. The QSO's goal at this meeting is to facilitate a conversation about the error that is blame free but helps the parties take responsibility and learn from the error. The process includes evaluating if the clinical site is a safe environment for students to learn.

At the end of the first year, the QSO disseminated the error and near-miss information as a formal presentation to the school of nursing faculty and nursing students at all levels. In addition, the QSO began developing partnerships with primary health care institutions by disseminating this reporting information. With just one year's results, the QSO increased visibility, provided safety education, made changes in reporting methods, and increased transparency in the school of nursing.

ONGOING ROLE

Currently, the QSO has an ongoing role in the school of nursing. Box 7.3 summarizes the QSO's activities. Evaluation of the QSO role is ongoing through surveys administered to faculty and students. Additional responsibilities may include the creation of a school of nursing safety council, dissemination of just culture information to faculty and students, development of a school of nursing safety newsletter, and close collaboration with adjunct faculty on reporting methods.

CONCLUSION

Increasing transparency in reporting errors and near misses may increase patient safety. Introducing safety early in a student's educational path may change the culture of reporting among nursing students and nurses at the bedside. Creating the role of a QSO was one attempt to bridge the safety gap in a school of nursing and assure transparency. Graduating nurses who have experienced transparency throughout their educational experience will be best equipped to apply those tools and knowledge to their practice.

References

Cooper, E. (2012). A spotlight on strategies for increasing safety reporting in nursing education. *The Journal of Continuing Education in Nursing, 43*(4), 162–168.

Cronenwett, L., Sherwood, G., Barnsteiner, J., Disch, J., Johnson, J., Mitchell, P., Sullivan, D., & Warren, J. (2007). Quality and safety education for nurses. *Nursing Outlook, 55*(3), 122–131.

Flynn, L., Liang, Y., Dickson, G., Xie, M., & Suh, D. (2012). Nurses' practice environments, error interception practices, and inpatient medication errors. *Journal of Nursing Scholarship, 44*(2), 180–186.

Hession-Laband, E., & Mantell, P. (2011). Lessons learned: Use of event reporting by nurses to improve patient safety and quality. *Journal of Pediatric Nursing, 26,* 149–155.

Howard, J. (2010). The missing link: Dedicated patient safety education within top-ranked US nursing school curricula. *Journal of Patient Safety, 6*(3), 165–171.

Institute of Medicine (IOM). (1999). *To err is human: building a safer health system.* Washington, DC: National Academy Press.

Institute of Medicine (IOM). (2001). *Crossing the Quality Chasm: A New Health System for the 21st Century.* Washington, DC: National Academy Press.

Karlsen, K., Hendrix, T., & O'Malley, M. (2009). Medical error reporting in America: A changing landscape. *Quality Management in Health Care, 18*(1), 59–70.

Kessels-Habraken, M., Van der Schaaf, T., De Jonge, J., & Rutte, C. (2010). Defining near misses: Towards a sharpened definition based on empirical data about error handling processes. *Social Science & Medicine, 70,* 1301–1308. doi:10.1016/j.socscimed.2010.01.006

Kurtzman, E., & Jennings, B. (2008). Trends in transparency: Nursing performance measurement and reporting. *The Journal of Nursing Administration, 38*(7), 349–354.

Lambton, J. & Mahlmeister, L. (2010). Conducting root cause analysis with nursing students: Best practice in nursing education. *Journal of Nursing Education, 49*(8), 444–448. doi:10.3928/01484834–20100430–03

Madden, I., & Milligan, F. (2004). Enhancing patient safety and reporting near misses. *British Journal of Midwifery, 12*(10), 643–647.

Paterick, Z., Paterick, B., Waterhouse, B., & Paterick, T. (2009). The challenges to transparency in reporting medical errors. *Journal of Patient Safety, 5*(4), 205–209.

Pauly-O'Neill, S. (2009). Beyond the five rights: Improving patient safety in pediatric medication administration through simulation. *Clinical Simulation in Nursing, 5*(5), 181–186.

Rowin, E., Lucier, D., Pauker, S., Kumar, S., Chen, J., & Salem, D. (2008). Does error and adverse event reporting by physicians and nurses differ? *Joint Commission on Accreditation of Healthcare Organizations, 34*(9), 537–545.

Sherwood, G. (2010). New views of quality and safety offer new roles for nurses and midwives. *Nursing and Health Sciences, 12,* 281–283.

Creating Partnerships

In *Achieving Excellence in Nursing Education* (Adams & Valiga, 2009), the National League for Nursing (NLN) defines a *partnership* as "an alliance between individuals or groups in which all parties mutually develop goals, collaborate to achieve those goals, and benefit from the alliance" (p. 184). In this section, we turn our focus to partnerships.

The NLN addresses partnerships in a number of its publications. In *Clinical Education in Prelicensure Nursing Programs,* Ironside and McNelis (2010) recommend that "new clinical models ... be developed and tested across sites, locations, types and programs, and levels of students," and that "these models ... foster partnerships among faculty, students, schools, clinical agencies, staff nurses and preceptors that align clinical learning with contemporary practice and health care needs" (p. 55).

Chapter 4 of the Institute of Medicine's 2011 report, *The Future of Nursing: Leading Change, Advancing Health* is titled "Transforming Education." This chapter, along with the recommendations of the publication, *A Summary of the February 2010 Forum on the Future of Nursing* (IOM, 2010), provides direction and guidance on many aspects of nursing education. The *Future of Nursing* calls on schools to expand students' knowledge of "culturally relevant care to meet the changing health needs of the U.S. population" and in areas outside the acute care setting (p. 190). This may be accomplished through partnerships with schools and practice settings. Nursing education programs can no longer work independently. In the current educational environment, nursing schools must work together "sharing resources to prepare the next generation of nurses" (IOM, 2011, p. 174). The *Forum on the Future of Nursing* also recommends that community colleges and universities develop partnerships.

In this section, Chapters 8 through 10 focus on partnerships and present examples of schools of nursing addressing this need for partnerships in learning among schools of nursing and with practice settings. To better meet the needs of patients, schools of nursing and practice settings must work more closely together to plan and implement curricula. One partnership form or model is the creation of a Designated Education

Unit (DEU), which requires faculty and staff to work closely together as they expand clinical education capacity in their work dedicated to educating future nurses.

Partnering activities are focused on educating nursing students with the end goal of improving patient outcomes. Various types of partnerships broaden the knowledge and experience base of students to effect quality patient outcomes. This section expands the discussion on partnerships by presenting ways that academia can partner among various educational institutions and with practice settings. The three chapters in this section provide evidence of the innovative capacity of nursing faculty as it applies to partnerships.

References

Adams, M. H., & Valiga, T. M. (2009). *Achieving excellence in nursing education.* New York: National League for Nursing.

Institute of Medicine (IOM). (2010) *A Summary of the February 2010 forum on the future of nursing.* Washington, DC: The National Academies Press.

Institute of Medicine (IOM). (2011). *The future of nursing: Leading change, advancing health.* Washington, DC: The National Academies Press.

Ironside, P. M., & McNelis, A. M. (2010). *Clinical education in prelicensure nursing programs.* New York: National League for Nursing.

8

The Clinical Faculty Role for a Dedicated Education Unit

Kelly M. Bower, PhD, RN, APHN-BC
Sandra M. Swoboda, MS, RN, FCCM
Pamela R. Jeffries, PhD, RN, FAAN, ANEF

Increased enrollments at schools of nursing and a clinical faculty shortage have created a need for change in clinical education (Murray, Crain, Meyer, McDonough, & Schweiss, 2010). The model of a Dedicated Education Unit (DEU) uses clinical nursing staff to integrate students into a clinical setting. Originating in Australia in the late 1990s, the DEU concept has been adopted by schools of nursing in New Zealand and the United States (Moscato, Miller, Logsdon, Weinberg, & Chorpenning, 2007; Mulready-Shick, Kafel, Banister, & Mylott, 2009). The model aims to:

1. Socialize students to the nurse role quickly and develop their sense of belonging

2. Help staff nurses develop in the preceptor role and advance their teaching skill

3. Encourage faculty to provide a mentor role and facilitate a community of learning on the unit

The model provides students with increased opportunities to practice skills, manage multiple patients, learn organization and prioritization, and become an integrated member of the health care team. However, this kind of innovative clinical nursing education requires a shift in the role of the clinical faculty member.

THE CLINICAL ACADEMIC PRACTICE PARTNERSHIP

In 2009, a private baccalaureate nursing program in the northeastern United States initiated a Clinical Academic Practice Partnership (CAPP) with two affiliate hospitals. Based on the concept of a DEU, CAPP maximizes expertise of staff nurses by actively engaging them in the education of students while delivering patient care (Edgecombe, Wotton, Gonda, & Mason, 1999; Bartz & Dean-Barr, 2003). The partner institutions were chosen based on existing affiliations, shared resources, and close geographic location. Nurse leaders from partner institutions were invited by the school of nursing to join an Executive Advisory Group and develop the new clinical model. BSN-prepared preceptors were identified by nurse managers on each unit, and the school of nursing provided a one-day workshop for preceptors to introduce the CAPP model and teaching strategies. Groups of six to eight students and one school of nursing faculty member were assigned to each CAPP unit. Each student was assigned a unit nurse preceptor with a student-to-preceptor ratio of either 1:1 or 2:1, depending on unit preference.

Although the CAPP model uses unit-based preceptors, it differs from the preceptor-ship and traditional clinical education models in many respects (Table 8.1). The CAPP model dedicates a unit, not just a single preceptor, to host students and to provide preceptors on an ongoing basis. The school of nursing provides close faculty mentorship of preceptors, and CAPP faculty members are present on the unit and meet with students and preceptors each clinical day. The CAPP model can be used for all levels of clinical placement from the first to the final semester. Additionally, CAPP faculty members serve as a resource for scholarship on CAPP units.

Faculty members in the CAPP model also assume different roles and responsibilities. In the traditional model, in which one clinical faculty oversees 8 to 12 students, students are often left waiting for faculty to deliver patient care. In the CAPP model, one preceptor oversees one or two students while those students care for all of the preceptor's assigned patients. CAPP faculty are still ultimately responsible for making sure that students meet course expectations; however, they do so by supporting the preceptor's teaching strategies and activities. The faculty member's primary role becomes that of mentor to the preceptor. In addition, CAPP faculty members act as a liaison between the unit and the school of nursing. Faculty who are accustomed to a role that focuses directly on students and patients may struggle with the shift to a unit- and preceptor-centered model.

RESPONSIBILITIES OF THE CAPP FACULTY

Responsibilities of CAPP faculty members can be divided into three broad categories: collaboration, guidance, and evaluation. In all of these areas, effective communication is essential for success.

School of nursing faculty must build strong collaborative relationships with the nurse manager, nurse educator, and charge nurse. Faculty should meet with these individuals quarterly to review the availability of the unit, learning needs of clinical preceptors, feedback from ongoing and prior rotations, and identification of new staff nurses as potential preceptors. Faculty must also apprise the manager, educator, and charge nurse of the students' level of clinical experience and expectations. Additionally, school of nursing faculty should serve as a resource to the staff for scholarship needs.

Collaboration between the CAPP faculty and school of nursing leadership helps to ensure a smooth launch of the initiative. Early in the implementation of CAPP, regularly scheduled meetings helped all parties review the intricacies involved in daily clinical management. Faculty shared challenges and brainstormed strategies for improvements with program leaders. For example, faculty were concerned that clinical experiences

TABLE 8.1

A Comparison of Traditional, CAPP, and Preceptorship Models of Nursing Education

	Traditional Model	CAPP Model	Preceptorship Model
Relationship with preceptor and unit	No preceptor. Faculty facilitates relationship with nurses and staff from clinical site.	Faculty closely mentor preceptors. Faculty meets regularly with nurse manager and engages in scholarly activities on unit. Faculty present on unit daily.	Faculty meets/talks with preceptor sporadically throughout clinical and may visit student and preceptor once during semester.
Patient assignments	Faculty select patient assignment for each student on a weekly basis.	Student works with the patients assigned to preceptor. Faculty helps preceptor identify patients most appropriate to meet student learning needs.	Student works with patients assigned to preceptor. No faculty input.
Expectation of student preparation	Prior to clinical, students look-up patient information to prepare for the clinical day.	Prior to first clinical day, faculty provide students with a list of common diagnoses and medications seen on the unit to look up and prepare. Just-in-time learning on the unit with preceptor.	Just-in-time learning with the preceptor.

(continued)

TABLE 8.1

A Comparison of Traditional, CAPP, and Preceptorship Models of Nursing Education (*Continued*)

	Traditional Model	CAPP Model	Preceptorship Model
Student instruction	Faculty directly supervise and teach students through provision of direct patient care. No preceptor. Faculty to student ratio is 1:6–12.	Faculty provide mentorship to preceptors in supervising and teaching students. Faculty debrief daily with students. Preceptor to student ratio 1:1 or 1:2, unit preference. Faculty to student ratio 1:6–12.	Faculty interact with students weekly via in-person or online group meetings for debriefing. Faculty to student ratio 1:12–15.
Daily routine	Faculty directly supervise students in provision of nursing care; this often leads to other students waiting for faculty and delays in patient care. Clinical occurs on designated clinical days.	Preceptors directly supervise students in provision of nursing care. No wait time for supervision and patients receive timely care. Faculty visit unit periodically throughout the day to check in with students and preceptors. Clinical occurs on designated clinical days.	Faculty have limited interaction with students at clinical sites. Clinical days based on preceptor schedule.
Evaluation of clinical skills	Skills performed under supervision of faculty and evaluated by faculty.	Skills performed under supervision of preceptor. Preceptor provides immediate feedback to student and written or verbal feedback to faculty.	Skills performed under supervision of preceptor. Preceptor provides immediate feedback to student and written or verbal feedback to faculty.

Written assignments	Faculty guide and grade written assignments.	Faculty guide and grade written assignments. On weeks students are developing care plans, faculty are available to meet with students to discuss the assignment.	Faculty guide and grade written assignments.
Final student evaluation	Faculty directly observe student performance and provide feedback to students.	Faculty are responsible for providing student evaluation. Evaluation incorporates preceptor evaluation of direct care and faculty debriefing.	Faculty are responsible for providing student evaluation. Evaluation is based on preceptor evaluation of direct care and faculty debriefing.
Relationship with the unit	Faculty and students are guests on the unit. Nurses and other staff have limited interaction with students.	Students become socialized to the unit, are integrated into the unit, and have extensive interaction with all members of the health care team. Faculty have strong relationship with unit staff and bridge relationships between the school of nursing and unit staff.	Students become socialized to the unit, are integrated into the unit, and have extensive interaction with all members of the health care team. Faculty liaison with nurse manager, educator, and preceptor as needed for student experience.

were not focused on specific course-related content; as a result, they developed a one-page weekly content review sheet that helped preceptors design clinical experiences to more specifically meet clinical objectives.

In the month prior to the start of a CAPP clinical rotation, faculty should establish good relationships, delineate clear lines of communication, and clarify expectations with the unit nurse preceptors. Our faculty began by visiting preceptors to introduce themselves and to review the clinical course, the level of student skill, and objectives for clinical learning, and to determine the preferred means and frequency of communication with preceptors. Once clinical began, weekly emails or letters to preceptors along with faculty presence on the unit provided effective preceptor guidance. Weekly written communication included a brief bulleted list of skills, assignments, and student objectives for the week to help preceptors select appropriate patients, target teaching, and adjust expectations. Students received a copy of these letters so that they were familiar with clinical expectations as well.

School of nursing faculty visibility on the unit and open lines of communication between faculty and preceptor were vital. Faculty found it helpful to be present at the beginning of the shift, which provided an opportunity to help direct the clinical experience, answer last-minute questions, and ensure that all assigned preceptors were present. In addition, faculty members were visible intermittently during the day to help foster a community of learning and provide preceptor mentorship. Preceptors often forgot that the reasoning behind their decisions or actions was not obvious or intuitive to the nursing student; preceptors thus were encouraged to think out loud regarding prioritizing, critical analysis, and decision making. Guidance was also provided on how to ask students questions that require critical thinking and an understanding of the larger clinical picture. Faculty helped preceptors identify appropriate educational activities for students and balance observational experiences with opportunities to provide direct care.

Faculty facilitated the student experience through course organization, regular debriefing, and encouraging students to take responsibility for their learning.

Methods for providing good course organization in the CAPP model are similar to that of the traditional clinical model. Regular debriefing can be done either in person or online. Although frequent debriefing is needed in the traditional model, it is even more essential in the CAPP model. Often students have questions that they are not comfortable asking their preceptor about patient care or unit functioning. In addition, debriefing allows students to process their feelings, to link course content to clinical experiences, and to think critically about clinical situations. It also provides faculty an opportunity to evaluate student performance.

CAPP faculty members encouraged students to take responsibility for their learning and empowered them to be appropriately assertive with their preceptors. For instance, if students are asked to perform a skill that they had not learned or practiced, they are instructed to tell their preceptor. This can be especially challenging for first-semester students. Faculty also helped students set learning goals with their preceptor, including opportunities to practice new skills and to build new knowledge.

Although CAPP faculty members do not supervise students at the bedside, they are responsible for student evaluation. Faculty members are solely responsible for grading student assignments, but all other student evaluation is a joint effort between the faculty and preceptor. We found it important to ask preceptors to provide written student evaluation on a regular basis. One method was to have preceptors rate students on a set of clinical behaviors each week. Evaluation forms were kept brief and simple to prevent overburdening the preceptors, but space for written narrative was included. When visiting the unit and talking to preceptors, we also asked preceptors explicit questions about student performance to determine specific areas in which students excelled or needed improvement.

CAPP faculty also made an effort to validate preceptor evaluation of student performance by asking students for patient reports and questioning them about pathophysiology, assessments, and interventions. Faculty questioned students about specific skills they practiced, how they performed, and their comfort level. They also asked students to review their progress toward self-directed education goals; to comment on the effectiveness of the relationship with their preceptor; and to explore the complexity of the health care environment, the nurse role, the student role, and their contribution to quality patient care.

CHALLENGES OF THE CAPP FACULTY ROLE

The biggest challenge for CAPP faculty members was adjusting to a hands-off approach toward student teaching and relying on preceptors to teach at the bedside. In the new role, faculty initially felt unsure of whether they were actively supporting student learning and found it hard to grasp the notion of being visibly invisible on the unit. Finding time for private, meaningful, face-to-face communication with busy preceptors was also difficult. We used a variety of strategies to overcome this challenge, including visits to the unit after students were gone, and visiting the unit in the afternoon, which tended to be less busy than in the morning.

Student evaluation was another challenge due to difficulties eliciting preceptor feedback. Solutions to this were similar to those previously discussed related to face-to-face communication with preceptors. Also, because faculty lacked direct interaction with patients, grading written assignments was initially difficult. This was easily resolved by getting faculty access to patient records.

Preceptor absences created another logistical challenge. Occasionally two students had to be assigned to one CAPP preceptor, or, with the help of the charge nurse, a non-CAPP preceptor was assigned a student. However, the program works best when nurses have been trained in the CAPP model. Training back-up preceptors will be vital to the program's long-term success.

CONCLUSION

In our experience, the key to ensuring a successful CAPP program is the dedication and commitment of all partner members. We had high-quality, cohesive clinical units that were motivated to mentor students and fostered an atmosphere of learning. Frequent opportunities for interaction and feedback between faculty, school of nursing administrators, unit administrators, and preceptors allowed faculty to evolve in their role and improve the program. CAPP faculty members were excited and committed to participating in this new, innovative educational model.

References

Bartz, C., & Dean-Barr, S. (2003). Reshaping clinical nursing education: an academic-service partnership. *Journal of Professional Nursing, 19,* 216–222. doi: 10.1016/S8755-7223(03)00090–5

Edgecombe, K., Wotton, K., Gonda, J., & Mason, P. (1999). Dedicated education units: a new concept for clinical teaching and learning. *Contemporary Nurse, 8,* 166–171. doi: 10.5172/conu.1999.8.4.166

Moscato, S. R., Miller, J., Logsdon, K., Weinberg, S., & Chorpenning, L. (2007). Dedicated education unit: an innovative clinical partner education model. *Nursing Outlook, 55,* 31–37. doi: 10.1016/j.outlook.2006.11.001

Mulready-Shick, J., Kafel, K. W., Banister, G., & Mylott, L. (2009). Enhancing quality and safety competency development at the unit level: an initial evaluation of student learning and clinical teaching on dedicated education units. *Journal of Nursing Education, 48,* 716–719. doi: 10.3928/01484834-20091113–11

Murray, T. A., Crain, C., Meyer, G., McDonough, M. E., & Schweiss, D. (2010). Building bridges: An innovative academic-service partnership. *Nursing Outlook, 58,* 252–260. doi: 10.1016/j.outlook.2010.07.004

Implementing Cultural Learning Activities through Community and Academic Partnerships: Introduction and Background

9

Joanne Noone, PhD, RN, CNE

Toni Bromley, MS, RN

Glenise McKenzie, PhD, RN

Sue Naumes, MSN, RN

Stephanie Sideras, PhD, RN

Heather Voss, MSN, RN

Preparing nurses to provide culturally competent care is a vital component of nursing education. Governmental and accrediting institutions for health care and nursing education all stress the importance of cultural competence in providing patient-centered care and addressing health disparities in diverse populations. Cultural competence is a component of the Patient-Centered Communication Standards currently being implemented for hospital accreditation by The Joint Commission (2010).

The US Department of Health and Human Services Office of Minority Health (2007) has developed national standards for culturally and linguistically appropriate services for health care. These standards include mandates for health care organizations receiving federal funds, guidelines for future mandates, and suggested recommendations for adoption by all health care agencies.

Both the American Association of Colleges of Nursing (AACN) and the National League for Nursing (NLN) include cultural competence as a core competency for undergraduate nurses. AACN (2008) has identified five key competencies related to cultural competence, and the concept of cultural competence is addressed in the core competency for nurses related to human flourishing identified by the NLN (2010).

This chapter describes two projects that brought together nursing faculty, clinical partners, and cultural consultants to develop cultural learning activities for an undergraduate curriculum. These projects were part of a two-year collaborative initiative in the northwest United States to support efforts to increase cultural competence in nursing and to identify promising practices for implementing cultural training programs. The initiative was spearheaded by the Oregon Center for Nursing and the Oregon Community Foundation. The initiative, called Nurturing Cultural Competence in Nursing (Oregon Center for Nursing, n.d.), was funded by the Robert Wood Johnson Foundation and the Northwest Health Foundation's Partners Investing in Nursing's Future program.

The faculty members involved in project development were from two partner baccalaureate and associate degree programs within the Oregon Consortium for Nursing Education (OCNE), a consortium of five baccalaureate and eight associate degree nursing

> # BOX 9.1 OCNE CORE COMPETENCIES THAT RELATE TO CULTURAL COMPETENCY
>
> A competent nurse practices relationship-centered care through the understanding that:
>
> - The effectiveness of nursing interventions and treatment plans depends, in part, on the attitudes, beliefs, and values of clients, which are influenced both by how professionals interact with clients and by the intervention itself.
> - Clients reflect the culture and history of their community and their broader population, and that these must be considered in developing nursing interventions.
>
> A competent nurse communicates effectively through the understanding that:
>
> - Successful communication requires attention to elements of cultural influences, variations in the use of language, and a participatory approach.
> - Effective health teaching requires being attuned to the clients' perspective, their previous understanding, and their ease of access to health information or degree of health literacy.

SOURCE: Oregon Consortium for Nursing Education, 2009.

programs throughout the state of Oregon. Partners share a three-year, competency-based curriculum with the first two years at the associate degree level and all three years occurring at the baccalaureate level. Cultural competency is reflected in the consortium's curricular core competencies, identified in Box 9.1.

PROJECT 1

Description

The first project was to develop online cultural competence tutorials focused on cultural assessment and reflective of Oregon's cultures. The project was initiated by the first author from the local baccalaureate program in partnership with representatives from a local health system. The representatives from the health system included a nursing practice leader and the head of nursing education as well as an employee in the health system's education department knowledgeable about their online learning system. Native American and Hispanic consultants were included on the project team to assist with tutorial review for cultural accuracy and to screen for bias and stereotyping. The Native American consultant was the head of Native American studies at the local university. The Hispanic consultant was a community leader and advocate who had a health care background as a respiratory therapist.

The project goals were:

1. To provide education and training in culturally and linguistically appropriate service delivery to current nursing students and nursing

faculty, and to licensed nursing staff and nonlicensed health care staff. This was measured by the number of students, faculty, and licensed and nonlicensed staff completing the tutorials.

2. As a result of completing the tutorials, to increase participants' knowledge of cultural beliefs and practices that may impact their clients' health beliefs, decisions, and practices. This was measured via participants' pre- and posttest knowledge scores based on tests developed for this project on cultural knowledge and awareness. A 10-question, multiple-choice pre- and posttest was developed for each module.

3. As a result of completing the tutorials, to increase participants' self-perceived cultural competence. This was measured by participants' pre- and posttest self-perceived cultural competency rating as measured on the Caffrey Cultural Competence in Healthcare Scale (CCCHS). This is a 28-item scale with established psychometric properties (Caffrey, Neander, Markle, & Stewart, 2005) to measure self-perceived knowledge, self-awareness, and comfort with skills of cultural competence. Each item has a rating of 1 to 5 (with 1 being less cultural knowledge, skill, etc., and 5 being most). Item scores are summed, with a mean of item scores providing a global score between 1 and 5.

Learning Modules

The three online, narrated modules that were developed provided continuing education credit for participants and are outlined below:

Module 1: Cultural Assessment

- Discuss general aspects of cultural beliefs and practices to incorporate into an assessment to determine their impact on health beliefs, decisions, and practices.

Module 2: Caring for the Hispanic Client

- Describe the changing ethnic demographics in Oregon.
- Discuss cultural beliefs and practices of Hispanic Americans that may impact their health beliefs, decisions, and practices.

Module 3: Caring for the Native American Client

- Describe the various Native American tribes in Oregon.
- Discuss cultural beliefs and practices of Native Americans that may impact their health beliefs, decisions, and practices.

Each module was separated into two sections for ease of completion. This was a recommendation made by representatives of the health care system to allow for short modules that could easily be completed during work time for employees.

TABLE 9.1		
Cultural Competency Project Participant Profile (N = 260)		
	Number	**Percent**
Nursing students	133	51
Nursing faculty	13	5
Registered nurses	65	25
Certified nursing assistants	23	9
Other personnel	26	10
Total	260	100

Project Outcomes

During the six-month study period, 260 students, faculty, and direct and indirect care providers completed all modules. Table 9.1 summarizes demographic data for participants. The 10 percent who were nonnursing direct and indirect care providers consisted of emergency, cardiac monitoring, imaging and radiology technicians; unit secretaries; and phlebotomists. All pretest measures occurred immediately before beginning Module 1; posttest measures were assessed at six weeks after completing all the modules. Pre- and posttest knowledge mean score changes are presented in Figure 9.1. All were significant at $p = .000$. CCCHS pre- and six-week posttutorial scores were available to compare for 60 participants. Paired t-test results showed mean scores improved from a 3.04 to 3.44 (significant at $p = .000$). Mean scores for individual items showed improvement for 20 of 28 items, with significant increase at $p < .05$ and none with a decrease (see Table 9.2).

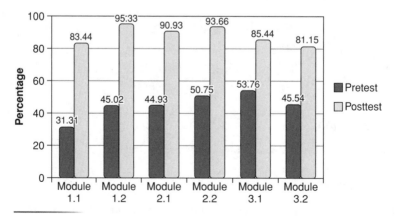

FIGURE 9.1 Mean knowledge scores for cultural competency project. N = 260, $p = .000$.

TABLE 9.2

Caffrey Cultural Competence in Healthcare[a] Inventory Items with Significant Increase ($p < .05$)

Item	Pretest	Posttest	P Value
How knowledgeable are you about the health care beliefs of a cultural group other than your own?	2.46	2.95	.000
How knowledgeable are you about the health care practices of a cultural group other than your own?	2.38	2.77	.000
How knowledgeable are you about the risk factors affecting the health status of a cultural group other than your own?	2.59	3.20	.000
How knowledgeable are you about the components of a comprehensive cultural assessment?	2.04	2.91	.000
How comfortable are you in doing a comprehensive cultural assessment on a client from a cultural group other than your own?	2.44	2.94	.004
How knowledgeable are you about the traditional foods of a cultural group other than your own?	2.67	3.18	.000
How comfortable would you be in working with a nonbiomedical folk healer to provide care to your client?	3.54	3.87	.028
How aware are you of the role of family members in the decision-making process regarding the health care of one of its members in a cultural group other than your own?	2.89	3.4	.001
How aware are you of the impact of your gender on your caregiving to clients from a culture other than your own?	2.96	3.56	.000
How comfortable are you in working with a cultural group other than your own to promote compliance with prescribed medical treatments in the context of their own cultural beliefs and practices?	3.45	4.09	.018
How comfortable are you in working with a cultural group other than your own when cultural beliefs and practices make compliance with prescribed medical treatments problematic?	2.66	3.14	.003
How knowledgeable are you about another culture's beliefs and practices related to dying and death?	2.2	2.93	.000

(*continued*)

TABLE 9.2

Caffrey Cultural Competence in Healthcare[a] Inventory Items with Significant Increase ($p < .05$) *(Continued)*

Item	Pretest	Posttest	P Value
How knowledgeable are you about another culture's beliefs and practices related to organ donation?	1.75	2.54	.000
How knowledgeable are you about another culture's beliefs around pregnancy and childbirth?	2.11	2.73	.000
How aware do you think you are about the influence on your caregiving of your own stereotypes regarding people from other cultures?	3.29	3.91	.000
How aware do you think you are regarding your own limitations in providing culturally competent care to a member of a cultural group other than your own?	3.45	4.09	.001
Overall, how would you evaluate your abilities to provide culturally competent care in the clinical setting to clients from a culture other than your own?	2.78	3.44	.000
How aware do you think you are about the impact of national policies on the health care of culturally diverse populations?	2.26	4.5	.000
How concerned are you about the impact of national policies on the healthcare of culturally diverse populations?	3.5	3.81	.014
How much influence do you think you can have on the formulation of national policies that impact the health of culturally diverse populations?	2.59	2.93	.011

[a]Rating on a scale of 1 to 5 (1 being less cultural knowledge, skill, etc., and 5 being most).

PROJECT 2

Description

The genesis for the second project occurred during evaluation of the first project. Discussions among faculty members took place about where to best place the tutorials for ongoing use in the curriculum. The need to develop additional cultural learning activities was identified by the faculty of the baccalaureate program. The local associate degree program partners students and faculty who also participated in completing the tutorials; a dialogue began with interested faculty from that program about intentionally developing and implementing a series of cultural learning activities throughout the undergraduate curriculum.

This second project sought to create (again with the assistance of cultural consultants) a series of didactic and clinical cultural learning activities to address different course outcomes within an undergraduate nursing program. All activities developed would be disseminated using an online faculty repository site accessible to more than 270 faculty at OCNE partner schools. Project faculty from both schools were invited to participate if they had an interest in the project goal and taught courses throughout the curriculum. Six faculty participated; four from the baccalaureate program and two from the associate degree partner school.

For year-one courses, the focus was on culturally appropriate health assessments and developing culturally appropriate plans of care. For year-two courses, the emphasis was on the cultural interpretation in acute and chronic illness and at the end of life. For year-three courses, the focus was on population health and health care delivery systems. Key indicators to measure project success were the number of cultural learning activities developed as a result of the project and the number of courses that had didactic and/or clinical cultural learning activities.

Outcomes

To start the projects, the six faculty met with the cultural consultants to discuss health-related objectives relevant to specific cultures and to plan learning activities specific to health-related areas. Project faculty intentionally designed active learning experiences such as case studies and simulations to contextualize cultural learning with better links between classroom and clinical learning, as recommended by Benner, Sutphen, Leonard, and Day (2009). Work was then undertaken individually by each faculty member to further develop learning activities.

The project team of faculty and consultants met after three months to present each of their learning activities and to provide feedback for further revision or adaptation. Fifteen cultural learning activities were identified and developed by the six project faculty. All of these were uploaded into the online learning repository.

These cultural learning activities span eight courses over the three-year curriculum and include a variety of learning strategies: Group presentations, scholarly papers, clinical learning activities, in-class case studies, PowerPoints®, and simulations (see Table 9.3 for selected learning activity examples for specific courses). Nine of the activities were for didactic, two were for simulation, and four were for clinical learning. The next academic year, these activities were implemented by the faculty team into the curriculum. A resource list for faculty across the consortium was also developed. Box 9.2 summarizes available cultural competency learning resources that faculty evaluated as useful during their development of learning activities. These can be used to enhance cultural learning activities.

USE OF CULTURAL CONSULTANT

A promising best practice from both of these projects was the use of cultural consultants to verify cultural learning activities while screening for bias and stereotyping.

TABLE 9.3

Selected Cultural Competency Learning Activities

Learning Activity	Description of Learning Activity	Evaluation and Recommendation
Poverty and Child Development First Year: Health Promotion	In preparation, students are to read two research-based studies that describe how poverty can impact typical childhood growth and development. The activity occurs in a Head Start preschool. The student must select a child to observe and compare that child's growth and development with typical growth and development as depicted in the text. Students are also asked to develop a 15-minute, age-appropriate health teaching session to be shared with the students and provide a simple flyer/coloring page describing the health topic covered to parents.	Students found the experience to be valuable. This activity provided the students with one more way to fine tune their assessment skills and begin to see the value of nurses in the community involved in health promotion. The students were well received by the children and teachers alike. Students must be cleared by a background check before being allowed to interact with the Head Start children. Recommendation: Plan at least two months in advance of your start date by getting all student paperwork and clearances to Head Start before beginning the activity.
World Culture Tour First Year: Health Promotion	This four-hour experiential/concept-based activity is designed to introduce the learner to common cultural beliefs and perspectives on health from four different ethnic groups. Each student is assigned to be an ambassador to one of the four selected cultures and learn about the culture during the first half of the session. Then students visit each table during the second half to learn about the different cultures.	This is an active learning activity that engages the learner. Student feedback has been positive: "I really enjoyed learning about the health beliefs of another culture—I never really thought about how different cultures regard health and what health means to them" (student comment). Recommendation: Students voiced that they would like more time with the activity and to learn about more cultures.
Hispanic Standardized Patient First Year: Chronic Illness	This simulation experience uses a live actor to bring a paper case study to life. The paper case is about a Hispanic migrant worker with undiagnosed diabetes. After working on the case in class, a standardized patient comes to class to be interviewed. All the students in the classroom are given the opportunity to meet the "client" and his interpreter.	By building on a paper case, the simulation provides students with practice identifying common points of intersection between the Hispanic culture and the culture of health care. The addition of an interpreter provides practice with both the strengths and challenges of communication through a third party.

Cultural Assessment Paper First Year: Acute Illness	Students care for a client and write a paper about how they would adapt care for this client if he or she was from another assigned culture. The client retains the same age, gender, and diagnosis.	This assignment works especially well in geographic regions with less diversity. Students can also learn about cultures not common within their locale. Students learn to consider how to adapt care and locate resources to help them.
Cultural Influences on Chronic Illness Second Year: Chronic Illness	This is a group activity to encourage students to explore cultural groups in relation to chronic illnesses and end-of-life expectations. The groups shared their learned information with the class via PowerPoints in class or posted on a shared website pamphlets, poster boards, fact sheets, skits, music, or guests demonstrating actual rituals and cleansing ceremonies.	Recommendations: Have instructor identify appropriate cultures. Provide additional verbal and written instructions to keep the students focused on how a nurse will interact with individuals; how a nurse could adapt the environment to aid the patient/client meet cultural needs. Include care of patient in the hospital, end-of-life expectations, cultural implications regarding health care education, and ability of the patient to adhere to recommendations.
Ethical and Cultural Considerations Related to Dementia Second Year: Chronic Illness	Written exercise based on a case study that includes issues relating to decision making and ethical considerations involving the care of a person with dementia and her caregiver. Students apply the Jonsen Model of Ethical Decision Making and modify their discussion of ethical issues and possible care plan based on an exploration of specific cultural factors. Students complete an analysis of the ethical and cultural considerations specific to the case study. This assignment can be modified to be a group activity and/or as a class discussion.	Students indicated the activity added to their learning in the course. Qualitative comments during class in reference to this assignment were all positive; they liked "having to think about how to change their approach to families based on culture."
Poverty Simulation Third Year: Populations Course	The Poverty Simulation used was designed by the Missouri Community Action Committee. The simulation includes families who attempt to live through one month of poverty by accessing traditional social service organizations, pawn shops, grocery stores, mortgage and utility companies, banks, day care centers, etc., to meet their families' needs.	The reaction of students and all participants was that of being exhausted and enlightened. Participants get a glimpse of what life might be like for families who live in poverty. This simulation takes a great deal of planning and training but is well worth it.

(continued)

TABLE 9.3

Selected Cultural Competency Learning Activities (Continued)

Learning Activity	Description of Learning Activity	Evaluation and Recommendation
Assessing Organizational Culture Third Year: Leadership Course	This concept-based activity invites learners to explore the culture of the organization or agency in which they are working within the context of healthy work environments and serves as a foundation for the Outcomes Improvement Project in the leadership course.	Feedback from students and faculty was positive: Students appreciated the opportunity to consider the culture of their organization and then share during a facilitated discussion. Students also felt that the activity was helpful in planning for change and how to best communicate within the organization.
Native American Powwow Clinical Experience Second or Third Year: Integrated Practicum	In preparation for this experience, students work in groups and identify the primary health risks of Native American populations. Each group picks a different health risk and builds a poster board and a flyer containing information on: 1. Who is at risk 2. Description and complications of the disease/illness 3. How to prevent the disease/illness 4. How to get help, contact information where one can find help locally The poster boards and flyers are presented to the public at the Native American Powwow, where students observe Native American culture and customs, provide first-aid booth, and perform simple health risk factor screenings.	Students were amazed at what they saw and experienced. The responses from students and from event participants were both very positive. Students were required to be present for one 4-hour period. Supplies needed: a simple first-aid kit, water, card tables, chairs, and a tent for shade.

BOX 9.2 FACULTY RESOURCES FOR CULTURAL LEARNING ACTIVITIES

American Association of Colleges of Nursing (AACN). (2008). Cultural competency in baccalaureate nursing education. www.aacn.nche.edu/Education/pdf/toolkit.pdf

- Toolkit with resource list and cultural learning activities

Garwick, A. (2009). *Getting to the heart of it: Ways to provide competent care of American Indian children and their families.* www.nursing.umn.edu/CCSHCN/ContinuingEd/WebModules/Module4-GettingtoHeart/Mod4Videos/home.html

- Video on how to provide patient-centered care to Native American clients

Grainger-Monsen, M., & Haslett, J. (2003). *Worlds apart: A four-part series on cross-cultural healthcare.* www.fanlight.com/catalog/films/912_wa.php

- Four vignettes with discussion guide on issues related to health care in four diverse populations

Kaiser Permanente Cultural Jeopardy Advanced Edition (n.d.). www.oregoncenterfornursing.org/index.php?mode=cms&pageId=diversity

- Cultural game for group activity

Kaiser Permanente Cultural Jeopardy Basic Edition (n.d.). www.oregoncenterfornursing.org/index.php?mode=cms&pageId=diversity

- Cultural game for group activity

Missouri Action Coalition Poverty Simulation (n.d.) http://communityaction.org/Poverty%20Simulation.aspx

- Three- to four-hour simulation that provides learners with an understanding of the impact of living in poverty

Rossiter, K., & Reeve, K. (2007). The Last Straw! A Board Game on the Social Determinants of Health©. www.thelaststraw.ca.

- Board game for group activity

Unnatural Causes: Is Inequality Making Us Sick? (2008). www.unnaturalcauses.org.

- A seven-part documentary series on health disparities with discussion guides and additional learning activities

US Department of Health and Human Services Office of Minority Health. (n.d.). *Think cultural health: Bridging the health care gap through cultural competency continuing education programs.* www.thinkculturalhealth.hhs.gov/

- Online continuing education that contains case studies that can be used for group discussions

For example, the cultural consultant assisted with setting a realistic background and patient presentation for the client in the Hispanic Standardized Patient discussed in Table 9.3 and provided dialogue in both Spanish and English. The result was a more realistic simulation. The simulation faculty member commented: "The cultural consultant brought the character to life. His work with the population of interest provided him the ability to help me with authentic dialogue for my simulation." Another faculty member stated: "I used the cultural consultant to review information I had found online related to end-of-life beliefs/customs. It was great to have an expert to confer with and to validate (or dispute) cultural information." Working with cultural consultants also had consequences beyond these projects. For example, we have invited cultural representatives from the community to sit on our school's community advisory board.

CONCLUSION

Sharing the vision of greater cultural competence in nursing education was and continues to be inspiring to faculty. They appreciated the collaborative efforts of the partnership and the support and opportunity to work with regional faculty and consultants. They all share a passion on the subject and valued the collegiality, dialogue, and action toward the shared commitment for client-centered, culturally competent health care. Faculty from both programs are currently collaborating on implementing the cultural learning activities across programs.

The learning activities have provided opportunities for nursing students to develop cultural competence. It is reassuring to witness the growth in cultural competence in students over time. Faculty members attribute this success to the focused and purposeful attention to concept development. Using the cultural competence learning activities with students has been very positive; their level of participation and interest in the topic has been enhanced by the use of a variety of activities (videos, reflection, written work, classroom discussions). As one faculty member stated: "The experience of developing learning activities that went across student levels was very positive for me as an educator. Taking a concept such as cultural competence and then figuring out how to best build learning experiences for our students (across our three-year program) makes my job more interesting and fun."

The projects discussed could be replicated elsewhere, although they may need to be adapted to the specific nursing curriculum and clinical experiences. Using partnerships to develop and implement learning activities can be mutually rewarding to all involved.

References

American Association of Colleges of Nursing (AACN). (2008). *Cultural competency in baccalaureate nursing education.* Retrieved from www.aacn.nche.edu/Education/pdf/toolkit.pdf

Benner, P., Sutphen, M., Leonard, V., & Day, L. (2009). *Educating nurses: A call for radical transformation.* San Francisco: Jossey-Bass.

Caffrey, R. A., Neander, W., Markle, D., & Stewart, B. (2005). Improving the cultural competence of nursing students: Results of integrating cultural content in the curriculum and an international immersion experience. *Journal of Nursing Education, 44*(5), 234–240.

National League for Nursing (NLN). (2010). *Outcomes and competencies for graduates of practical/vocational, diploma, associate degree, baccalaureate, master's, practice doctorate, and research doctorate programs in nursing.* New York: Author.

Oregon Center for Nursing (n.d.). *Nurturing cultural competence in nursing.* Retrieved from http://www.ocnnursingdiversity.org/ index.php?mode=cms&pageId=NCCN

Oregon Consortium for Nursing Education (OCNE). (2009). *Curriculum competencies.* Retrieved from http://ocne. org/Curriculum%20Competency%20 May%202009.pdf

The Joint Commission (2010). Advancing effective communication, cultural competence, and patient- and family- centered care. Retrieved from www.jointcommission.org/Advancing_ Effective_Communication/

US Department of Health and Human Services Office of National Minority Health (2007). *National standards on culturally and linguistically appropriate services.* Retrieved from http:// minorityhealth.hhs.gov/templates/ browse.aspx?lvl=2&lvlID=15

10

The Impact of International Leadership Development:
A Shared Nursing Educational Service-Learning Partnership

Sharon Elizabeth Metcalfe, EdD, RN

The nursing profession will be facing a worldwide shortage of practicing nurses, as well as nursing leaders, by the year 2020 (Aiken, Cheung, & Olds, 2009; Buerhaus, Auerbach, & Staiger, 2007). The current workforce consists of an aging nursing population, primarily baby boomers. In 2013, one third of the United States' nursing workforce is reported to now be 50 years of age and above (Health Resources and Services Administration, 2013). Despite tremendous efforts by the US government to provide funding for increasing the number of nurses and improving environmental work conditions, health care is forecasted to enter a period called "Xtreme nursing," with marked imbalance between the supply of and demand for nurses (Johnson, Billingsley, & Costa, 2006). With the emerging global retirement of clinical nursing care providers, university faculty, and nursing administrators, it is imperative that the profession of nursing prepare its workforce to develop into the next generation of nursing leaders.

This chapter describes an innovative collaborative international partnership focused on leadership development. The goal was to develop future nursing leaders (RN-to-BSN undergraduate students) through preparation and delivery of shared service-learning health care presentations. Clinical presentations were conducted by American nursing professionals in hospital, outpatient, and community care settings in Scotland, England, and Wales.

THE CALL FOR TRANSFORMATION OF THE NURSING PROFESSION

The 2011 report by the Institute of Medicine (IOM), "The Future of Nursing: Leading Change, Advancing Health," calls for nurses to practice at the full extent of their education and achieve higher academic degrees through seamless academic progression. Currently, 65 percent of the nation's nurses hold associate degrees; the report calls for 80 percent of RNs to achieve a bachelor of science degree or higher by the year 2020 (IOM, 2011). Nurses need to become instrumental in redesigning health care and information data collection (American Nurses Association [ANA], 2010). The Tri-Council for Nursing, which includes the American Association of Colleges of Nursing (AACN), the ANA, the American Organization of Nurse Executives (AONE), and the National League for Nursing (NLN), is united in supporting these recommendations (Tri-Council for Nursing, 2010).

The IOM report emphasizes the need to prepare nurses to lead change in advancing health (IOM, 2011). This pivotal recommendation states that nursing educational programs, nursing leaders, and health care decision makers must ensure that nurses are full partners in leadership decisions (IOM, 2011). Effective nursing leaders create positive and supportive work environments with improved nursing job satisfaction, increased productivity, and marked increases in retention of staff, and by fostering organizational commitment (Kowalski, 2009).

Developing future nursing leaders from today's clinical practicing nurse workforce requires coaching and mentoring. Seasoned leaders must provide guided direction to staff nurses to help them acquire the challenging skills needed for leading today's health care organizations (Metcalfe, 2010). The International Council of Nurses (ICN), a federation of 130 national nursing associations that represents 13 million nurses, has recognized the need for increasing nursing leadership through its Global Nursing Leadership Institute. The institute's focus is for senior nursing leaders worldwide to seek mutual nursing practice approaches in addressing world health care issues (ICN, 2010). Smith (2006) has called for nursing leaders in the United States and abroad to address the leadership needs for improvements in health care through refocusing nursing curricula to include global health. The need for knowledgeable and educated nursing leaders will be paramount for the emerging global health care environment of the next decade. The time to prepare a new generation of nursing leaders is now.

LITERATURE REVIEW OF INTERNATIONAL NURSING EDUCATIONAL PARTNERSHIPS

Transcultural nursing care and exploration has been a cornerstone of nursing since the formative classic work of Leininger (1999). Broadening of the global diversity perspective allows an increase in leadership development and preparation (Schim, Doorenbois, & Borse, 2005).

The Sigma Theta Tau International Honor Society of Nursing encourages international educational exposure (Sullivan, 2008), and sponsors and promotes annual programs that promote international nursing collaborations. International educational collaborations allow linking of leadership opportunities, learning of advocacy roles, and fostering of ethical accountability (Leppa & Terry, 2004). Educational collaborations undertaken by the author as well as multiple nursing groups demonstrate that international exposure increases understanding of global nursing care perspectives, awareness of cultural sensitivity, and empowerment among nursing colleagues across national boundaries (Foster, 2009; Gerrish, 2004; Bennet & Holtz, 2008).

A multitude of volunteer organizations promote cultural exchange and awareness. Opportunities exist with the United Nations Children's Fund (UNICEF), People to People Ambassadors, and Project Hope. A variety of programs exist that offer hands-on clinical care and diversity through team methods (Lindahl, Dagborn, & Nilsson, 2008; Kuehn, Chircop, Downe-Wamboldt, et al., 2005).

During the last decade, a plethora of international nursing collaborations has emerged. San Francisco State University's school of nursing program initiated programs for students to travel to Italy, Peru, Thailand, Ghana, and the United Kingdom, providing students with exposure to differences and similarities in family-centered care (Perry & Mander, 2005). Johns Hopkins University formed a partnership with Haiti Medical Mission to provide health care services to the poor of Leon, Haiti (Sloand & Groves, 2005). The purpose was for Haitian practitioners to demonstrate culturally sensitive care and educate the visiting American nursing students through the comparisons and contrasts in illnesses.

Some international nursing educational collaborations have focused on leadership development through direct nursing care in service-learning initiatives. Jacoby (1996) first described service-learning as experiential education that used structured opportunities to address human and community needs designed to promote student learning and development through reflection and reciprocity. With service-learning education, every individual, entity, and organization functions as both a teacher and a learner, and participants are seen as colleagues (Laplante, 2009). Additional benefits of service-learning include team building, initiating collaborative relationships with others, and developing leadership skills of negotiation, accountability, and social responsibility (Baumberger-Henry, Krouse, & Borucki, 2006). Service-learning international programs have been primarily implemented to provide clinical or direct nursing care to patients in developing nations (Axley, 2009; Bentley & Ellison, 2007; Callister & Cox, 2006; Wittman-Price, Anselmi, & Espinal, 2010). Through these collaborations, nurses have become knowledgeable concerning the disparities of the world's most at-risk populations (Chinn, 2005). Students have reported experiencing personal transformations as a result of service-learning experiences with diverse populations (Worrell-Carlisle, 2005).

INTERNATIONAL NURSING LEADERSHIP PARTNERSHIP CONCEPTUAL FRAMEWORK

McAuliffe and Cohen (2005) conducted a comprehensive literature review of 79 articles related to international nursing education and research programs in developed and developing countries (1982–2003). Based on their review, they recommended that future international educational nursing leadership service-learning partnerships have as their foundation a conceptual framework based on the model "Engaging Tomorrow's International Nursing Leaders" (Garner, Metcalfe, & Hallyburton, 2009). This concept model presents nursing practice as encouraging patient advocacy, seeking accountability for patients and their care, and becoming activist leaders for clients and families (Garner, Metcalfe, & Hallyburton, 2009).

Using the three components of the model (advocacy, accountability, and activism), nurses from the United States have delivered service-learning presentations on topics of international health concerns at both clinical and university sites within the United Kingdom. Through the process of presenting clinical presentations, the nurses grew in their leadership skills and role development as future nursing leaders.

THE INTERNATIONAL NURSING LEADERSHIP EDUCATIONAL PARTNERSHIP

Since the fall of 2007, a program for undergraduate RN-to-BSN nurses to develop as future nursing leaders has been offered with a southeastern regional comprehensive university school of nursing in the United States in association with various universities and hospitals in the United Kingdom. Each partnership was initiated through a year-long process of determining mutual goals for conducting a successful program. Administrative and academic leadership provided annual financial stipend of support for the southeastern regional comprehensive university and the universities and hospitals in the United Kingdom (Scotland, England, and Wales).

History of the International Nursing Leadership Educational Partnership

The foundation for the current program began in 1999 with a pilot program that included a year of planning with three university schools of nursing located in the United Kingdom. The pilot program included 17 faculty and students; its objective was for participants to become culturally aware of health care delivery systems, specifically the differences and similarities between the National Health Trust in the United Kingdom and the managed health care system in the United States. Precourse surveys assessing student knowledge of health care systems were administered and revealed that 98 percent of the participants had minimal understanding. Postcourse evaluation student surveys indicated a marked improvement in knowledge acquisition. To the survey question, "Did you acquire a new level of understanding of the health systems within the United Kingdom as compared to the USA?" the students responded overwhelmingly with a 100 percent marked increase in knowledge gain. The pilot program thus met its primary objective.

Goals of the International Nursing Leadership Educational Partnership

In 2005, the program's objective changed from having the RN-to-BSN students describe the unique health care systems of both countries to a new objective of demonstrating leadership skills through service-learning presentations. Simultaneously, the educational partnership was expanded to incorporate a new leadership focus. The goal of these changes was to create opportunities for future leadership roles through formal service-learning presentations for developing RN-to-BSN nursing students. The modified program would provide an international setting for both leadership development and collaborative dialogue through knowledge dissemination of global health care issues.

Service-learning presentations have included such topics as the status of national health care reform in the United States as compared with the National Health Service within the United Kingdom, health care of chronic illnesses such as heart disease, and specialty population care issues such as rising rates of diabetes. Additional presentations have included the approaches to nursing care internationally in regional health care facilities, and the myriad of educational pathways for professional nurses on both continents.

Program Logistics and Preparation

In total, 38 RN-to-BSN students have participated in the annual program, which has been conducted as part of 8 days of leadership development activities within the United Kingdom. Participants additionally toured health care facilities to observe nursing care in three regions in the United Kingdom.

In 2005, to minimize travel costs for participants, the program began using the services of a nationally recognized educational student travel company. The travel specialists guided the coordination of scheduling flights, ground transportation, lodging, and meals. This allowed the program nursing educators to focus their energies on mentoring the nursing student participants for their service-learning presentations.

Mutual Benefits of International Nursing Leadership Partnerships

The primary academic goal of the international partnerships was to provide a global opportunity for RN-to-BSN students to demonstrate their developing leadership skills through formal presentation of nursing care practices in an international setting. The secondary goal was to disseminate what was learned to practicing nurses, nursing students, and a variety of health care professionals within the United Kingdom.

The school of nursing at each of the participating universities annually utilized qualitative and quantitative methods for assessing the impact of the service-learning presentations. Faculty from each of the universities in the United Kingdom reported a satisfaction level of 100 percent for participant reactions to the presentations and shared dialogue on mutual health care concerns. Qualitative responses with the United Kingdom participants indicated that having dialogue with their visiting nursing peers had a significant impact and increased their understanding of clinical nursing care within the United States.

In the United States, evaluative surveys focused questions on leadership development and were distributed to the 38 student participants. RN-to-BSN students who participated from 2005 through 2010 evaluated the experience as having made a pivotal impact on both their professional and personal lives. These positive evaluations are reflected

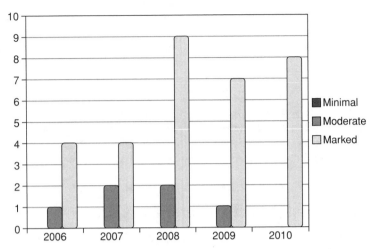

Did you develop new leadership skills in presenting nursing trends to professional peers in the United Kingdom and the United States?

FIGURE 10.1 Leadership skills acquisition survey responses from American RN-to-BSN students who participated in *the International Nursing Leadership Educational Partnership* program from 2005 through 2010.

in responses to three specific postsurvey questions administered to the students that focused on the development of new leadership skills (Fig. 10.1), the strengthening of leadership skills (Fig. 10.2), and the sharing of leadership skills with others (Fig. 10.3). Qualitative responses noted that participants appreciated the opportunity to travel to the United Kingdom and have the honor of presenting internationally.

Additionally, the visiting RN-to-BSN students recorded their impressions of the leadership development experience via journaling. Intensive student reflective journaling was used to assess their perspectives of the program. Students wrote extensively about their experiences with nurses and students in the United Kingdom, and analyzed the quality of their presentations and their impact on their nursing peers in the United Kingdom.

Qualitative themes from the reflective journals centered on the broadening awareness of the health care systems and nursing professional roles within the United Kingdom and the United States. Additional themes focused on the contrasting pathways for nursing education. Visiting RN-to-BSN students held the perception that nursing in the United Kingdom provided a more holistic approach to nursing care to clients in inpatient and outpatient settings. Further reflective themes included the perception that patients in the United Kingdom received increased nursing attention with total patient care, spiritual needs, and emotional well-being. Nurses were found to focus more on the patient and spend less time on technology as a professional nurse.

After returning to the United States, the RN-to-BSN students presented their reflections to their coworkers at their places of employment. These facilities included home health care agencies, hospitals, schools, community care sites, and other facilities of

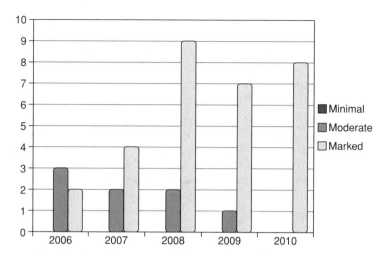

Did you strengthen your nursing leadership skills in your current workplace as a result of this learning experience?

FIGURE 10.2 Strengthening leadership skills survey responses from American RN-to-BSN students who participated in *the International Nursing Leadership Educational Partnership* program from 2005 through 2010.

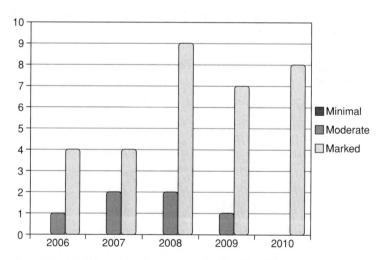

Did you increase your interest in sharing your leadership skills/mentoring role in the future?

FIGURE 10.3 Sharing and mentoring leadership skills survey responses from American RN-to-BSN students who participated in *the International Nursing Leadership Educational Partnership* program from 2005 through 2010.

nursing care provision. This dissemination activity helped to further their leadership role development through delivery of their experiences to peers at their home agencies. Since returning to the United States, each of the students has been promoted to a nursing leadership position in his or her home institution.

Through their accomplishments of successfully presenting to international colleagues, the participating RN-to-BSN students reported that they had increased confidence in their potential abilities to lead others. Additionally, they felt empowered to present their experiences and new knowledge to their coworkers and supervisors at their home work environments in the United States. The international leadership educational partnership experience has left lifetime impressions on the RN-to-BSN students. The RN-to-BSN students have grown professionally. The students, nurses, and academic faculty within the United Kingdom have expressed similar positive outcomes.

RECOMMENDATIONS FOR FUTURE INTERNATIONAL LEADERSHIP PARTNERSHIPS

The International Nursing Leadership Partnerships has developed three recommendations for future nursing educators interested in program replication:

1. Shared nursing student service-learning experiences strengthen the academic bonds between universities and clinical facilities on an international level.

   Recommendation: Increasing the number of international nursing academic and clinical partnerships will promote the understanding of mutual global health care issues.

2. Developing the groundwork for international academic nursing student service-learning presentations creates leadership development opportunities through communication and scholarly dissemination.

   Recommendation: Increasing international partnerships creates long-lasting educational bonds. Partnership programs provide a vehicle for meeting the emerging need for nurses to lead into the next decade.

3. Recommendations for replication of this program include:
   - Develop initial mutual objectives with overseas partners.
   - Seek the expert guidance of an educational travel company.
   - Structure personal safety trip precautions with participants.
   - Plan program one year in advance for student payment plans.
   - Provide for mentoring and rehearsal of student presentations.
   - Develop pre- and postevaluative surveys to assess learning.
   - Provide opportunities for clinical dialogue with all participants.
   - Offer pre- and posttrip debriefing sessions with participants.
   - Allow social time for students to interact with peers overseas.
   - Recognize contributions of partners with appreciation letters.

References

American Association of Colleges of Nursing (AACN). (2010). AACN reports continued increase in BSN enrollment. Retrieved from http://news.nurse.com/article/20101201/NATIONAL02/112060066

American Nurses Association (ANA). (2010). ANA applauds IOM's release of 'Future of Nursing' report. Retrieved from http://www.nursingworld.org/MainMenue Categories/The Practice of Professional Nursing/workplace/IOM-Future-of-Nursing Report 1/IOM-Report.aspx

Aiken, L.H., Cheung, R.B, & Olds, D. M. (2009). Education policy initiatives to address the nurse shortage in the United States. *Health Affairs, 28*(4), 646–656. doi:10.1377/hlthaff.28.4.w646

Axley, L. (2009). Nursing in diverse cultures: An international experience. *Tennessee Nurse, 72*(1), 4–5.

Baumberger-Henry, M. L., Krouse, A. M., & Borucki, L. C. (2006). Giving and receiving: A case study in service learning. *Nurse Educator, 31*(6), 249–252.

Bennet, D., & Holtz, C. (2008). Building cultural competence: A nursing practicum in Oaxaca, Mexico. In C. Holtz (Ed.), *Global Health Care: Issues and policies* (pp. 601–614). Boston, MA: Jones and Bartlett.

Bentley, R., & Ellison, K. J. (2007). Increasing cultural competence in nursing through international service-learning experiences. *Nurse Educator, 32*(5), 207–211. doi: 10.1097/01.NNE.0000289385.14007.b4

Buerhaus, P. I., Auerbach, D. I., & Staiger, D. O. (2007). Recent trends in the registered nurse labor market in the US: Short-run swings on top of long-term trends. *Nurse Economics, 25*(2), 59–66.

Callister, L. C., & Cox, A. H. (2006). Opening our hearts and minds: The meaning of international clinical nursing electives in the personal and professional lives of nurses. *Nursing & Health Sciences, 8*(2), 95–102.

Chinn, P. (2005). Nursing activism and scholarship to address health disparities. *Advances in Nursing Science, 28*(3), 193.

Foster, J. (2009). Cultural humility and the importance of long-term relationships in international partnerships. *The Journal of Obstetrics, Gynecology, and Neonatal Nursing, 38,* 100–107. doi. 10.1111/j.1552-6909.2008.00313.x

Garner, B. L., Metcalfe, S. E., & Hallyburton, A. (2009). International collaboration: A concept model to engage nursing leaders and promote global nursing education partnerships. *Nurse Education in Practice, 9,* 102–108.

Gerrish, K. (2004). The globalization of the nursing workforce: Implications for education. *International Nursing Review, 51,* 65–66.

Health Resources and Services Administration. (2013). The U.S. nursing workforce trends in supply and education. Health Resources and services administration. Bureau of Health Professions National Center for Workforce Analysis Report. April 2013. (p. vii).

Institute of Medicine (IOM). (2011). The future of nursing: Leading change, advancing health. Robert Wood Johnson Foundation Initiative on the Future of Nursing at the Institute of Medicine. Retrieved from www.iom.edu/Reports/2010/The-Future-of-Nursing-Leading-Change-Advancing-Health.aspx

International Council of Nurses (ICN). (2010). ICN–Burdett global nursing leadership institute. Retrieved from www.icn.ch/pillarsprograms/global-nursing-leadership-institute/

Jacoby, B. (1996). Service-learning in today's higher education. In B. Jacoby (Ed.), *Service Learning in Higher Education* (pp. 3–5). San Francisco, CA: Jossey-Bass.

Johnson, J. E., Billingsley, M. C., & Costa, L. L. (2006). Xtreme nursing and the nursing shortage. *Nursing Outlook, 54*(5), 294–299.

Kowalski, K. (2009). Nursing workforce of the future. *Perioperative Nursing Clinics, 2*(4), 265–272.

Kuehn, A., Chircop, A., Downe-Wamboldt, B., Sheppard-LeMoine, D., Murnaghan, D., Elliott, J., Critchley, K., et al. (2005). Exploring nursing roles across North American borders. *The Journal of Continuing Education in Nursing, 36*(4), 153–162.

Laplante, N. (2009). Discovering the meaning of reciprocity for students engaged in service-learning. *Nurse Educator, 34*(1), 6–8.

Leininger, M. M. (1999). Transcultural nursing: An imperative for nursing practice. *Imprint, 46*(5), 50–52, 61.

Leppa, C., & Terry, L. (2004). Reflective practice in nursing ethics education: International collaboration. *Journal of Advanced Nursing, 48*(2), 195–202.

Lindahl, B., Dagborn, K., & Nilsson, M. (2008). A student-centered clinical educational unit-description of a reflective learning model. *Nurse Education in Practice, 9*(1), 5–12. doi: 10.1016/j.nepr.2008.03.008.

McAuliffe, M. S., & Cohen, M. Z. (2005). International nursing research and educational exchanges: A review of the literature. *Nursing Outlook, 53*(1), 21–25.

Metcalfe, S. E. (2010). Educational innovation: Collaborative mentoring for future nursing leaders. *The Journal of Creative Nursing: A Journal of Values, Issues, Experiences & Collaboration. 16*(4), 168–171.

Perry, S., & Mander, R. (2005). Quick reads. A global frame of reference: Learning from everyone, everywhere. *Nursing Education Perspectives, 26*(3), 148–151.

Schim, S., Doorenbois, A. Z., & Borse, N. (2005). Cultural competence among Ontario and Michigan healthcare providers. *Journal of Nursing Scholarship, 37*(4), 354–360.

Sloand, E., & Groves, S. (2005). A community-oriented primary care nursing model in an international setting that emphasizes partnerships. *Journal of the American Academy of Nurse Practitioners, 17*(2), 47–50.

Smith, B. A. (2006). The role of nursing leaders in global health issues and global health policy. *Nursing Outlook, 54*(6), 309–310.

Sullivan, E. J. (2008). *Effective leadership and management in nursing: International edition.* Upper Saddle River, NJ: Prentice Hall.

Tri-Council for Nursing, (2010). Tri-Council for Nursing Calls for Collaborative Action in Support of the IOM's *Future of Nursing* Report. Retrieved from www.nursingworld.org/MainMenuCategories/ThePracticeof ProfessionalNursing/workplace/IOM-Future-of-Nursing-Report_1/Tri-Council-PR-IOM-Report.aspx

Wittman-Price, R. A., Anselmi, K. K., & Espinal, F. (2010). Creating opportunities for successful international student service-learning experiences. *Holistic Nursing Practice, 24*(2), 89–98. doi: 10.1097/HNP.0b013e3181d3994a

Worrell-Carlisle, P. J. (2005). Service learning: A tool for developing cultural awareness. *Nurse Educator, 30*(5), 197–202.

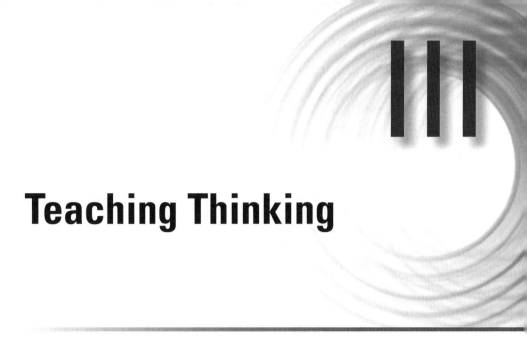

Teaching Thinking

The Institute of Medicine report, *The Future of Nursing: Leading Change, Advancing Health* (IOM, 2011) advises nursing programs to identify core competencies students will achieve by the time they complete the program of study.

> "The value of competency-based education in nursing is that it can be strongly linked to clinically based performance expectations. It should be noted that 'competencies' here denotes not task-based proficiencies but higher-level competencies that represent the ability to demonstrate mastery over care management knowledge domains and that provide a foundation for decision-making skills under a variety of clinical situations across all care settings" (IOM, 2011, p. 200).

The Future of Nursing recommends that nursing programs incorporate a core competency that promotes the students' abilities in clinical judgment and critical thinking. The report bases some of its recommendation on the publication *Educating Nurses: A Call for Radical Transformation* (Benner et al., 2010). In presenting important lessons on thinking from Benner's research, *The Future of Nursing,* quoting from Benner:

> " … calls for teaching that invites students to develop a sense of salience, clinical reasoning, and clinical imagination. To achieve this, the best teachers must teach well beyond disembodied content, teaching students instead how to *be* a nurse who uses evidenced-based knowledge and cultivates habits of thinking for clinical judgment and skilled knowhow. Their (the best teachers') teaching is integrative and patient-centered … these teachers coach their students, engaging them in experiential learning to develop situated knowledge, skills, and ethical comportment." (p. 552)

Safe, quality nursing care is possible only if the nurse knows how to think. Teaching thinking is not an easy task and requires teaching/learning approaches that may be quite different than what are typically used in nursing programs. Students must no longer be passive attendees during class sessions, but rather active participants in all learning environments, engaging not only in learning content but using the content the way a nurse uses the content. In this section, Chapters 11 through 18 provide examples of innovative strategies that teach not just content, but also thinking in the classroom, simulation laboratory, and clinical setting.

References

Institute of Medicine (IOM). (2011). *The future of nursing: Leading change, advancing health.* Washington, DC: The National Academies Press.

Benner, P., Sutphen, M., Leonard, V., & Day, L. (2010). *Educating nurses: A call for radial transformation.* San Francisco: Jossey-Bass.

11

Deepening Learning in Foundational Skills:
Visual Thinking Network Strategy

Kristen A. Sethares, PhD, RN, CNE
Kathryn L. Gramling, PhD, RN

Nursing is both science and art—thinking and doing. Students of nursing are being prepared to provide safe patient care with knowledge and skill in complex, technological, and poignant human predicaments. Educators strive to design curricula that emphasize essential "core" knowledge and skills while broadening the undergraduate's understanding about the multifaceted experience of caregiving.

One foundational skill in nursing is the use of aseptic technique. Numerous concepts are synthesized and demonstrated in the production of a skill. For example, the knowledge underlying the use of aseptic technique involves concepts of microbiology, pathophysiology, anatomy, safety, and wound healing, among others. When students comprehend the knowledge elements at work in such a skill, they may better adapt appropriately in diverse practice situations.

There is little evidence that traditional teaching methods have, in fact, helped students integrate conceptual learning with skill acquisition. Frequently, a type of "show and tell" is employed for skill learning. Students usually have the opportunity to witness the skill (either in person or by video), and are provided with a procedural checklist to memorize and emulate in a return demonstration (Craven & Hirnle, 2009). In a spirit of searching for best practices and in an era of evolving cognitive science, nurse educators must explore the efficacy of traditional models and new methods for skill learning.

This chapter describes the testing of an innovative strategy to promote the integration of thinking and doing (concept and procedure) in learning a basic skill: aseptic technique. Understanding the particular concepts involved in asepsis, creatively depicting those concepts, and linking them in a meaningful way through a Visual Thinking Network (VTN) may advance the nature and depth of the student's knowledge. This study applies a strategy that is guided by the latest neurocognitive theory of learning and has been demonstrated to be effective in earth science education.

INNOVATIVE PEDAGOGY

The authors were inspired by a presentation given by James Zull through the Office of Faculty Development at University of Massachusetts, Dartmouth. Zull is a biologist, educator, and author of *The Art of Changing the Brain* (2002). He argues that the structure and function of the brain can be the teacher's ally. Zull superimposes the cerebral cortex of the brain onto Kolb's learning cycle to show where experiences are sensed, reflected on, integrated, formed, and tested. Sensory experience comes from outside the brain of the student, but the student does something with that experience (Zull, 2002). Zull writes that knowledge is not only stored in brain cells (neurons), but is created when neurons are built upon and extended. "Neuronal networks are knowledge" (Zull, 2002, p. 92) and, therefore, learning occurs by building on existing neuronal networks or previous knowledge.

Dr. Palma Longo, an educator and biologist, developed and tested a new active learning strategy, Visual Thinking Networks (VTN), which facilitates the development of neuronal networks. Longo, Anderson, and Wicht (2002) depict the VTN as a "knowledge representation strategy" (2002, p. 3) that builds neuronal networks during learning. The VTN serves to "represent, organize and revise her/his meaning making of science knowledge by chunking and linking conceptual labels with symbolic visualizations of scientific concepts, processes, and experiences into a coherent whole (p. 3)." Students construct a two-dimensional illustration on paper using forms, images, shapes, color, words, and associations as they build their understanding.

The VTN employs foundational neurocognitive principles, processes, and goals. The student creates meaning through activating multiple sensory perceptions and expressions. A VTN is imaginative, builds on prior knowledge, and does not need to be hierarchical. With a VTN, "the learners make their knowledge explicit in a highly meaningful and idiosyncratic form" (Longo, 2007). Color is added because "neurocognitively color is a form of knowledge in our brain" (Longo, 2007, p. 1).

Two studies have demonstrated the effective use of the VTN strategy in earth science education (Longo et al., 2002; Longo, 2007). In a controlled experimental study, 56 ninth graders were randomized into three groups, pretested for earth science knowledge, and provided the same earth science lecture and laboratory by the same instructor; however, they were given three different learning strategies. The control group was given a writing strategy. The two experimental groups used either black and white or color VTN. Significant differences were found in pre- and posttest knowledge between the groups, with the highest achievement in the group using color VTN (Longo et al., 2002). Further, another pre–post randomized, controlled study (Longo, 2007) with 140 teenagers found a significantly higher achievement in science knowledge for females who used color in VTNs when compared to males. Color in VTNs enhanced long-term problem solving for females. The present pilot project describes the first utilization of color VTN in promoting skill knowledge in nursing education.

CONSTRUCTING A VTN

Longo (2007) developed a guide for students to use in constructing their network. It includes using a list of teacher-generated concepts important to the understanding of a major knowledge principle. From the concept list, students choose one central concept

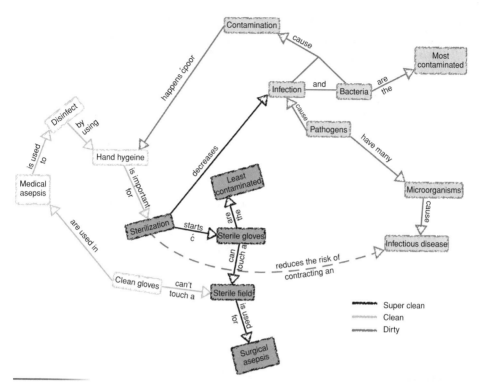

FIGURE 11.1 A student's VTN. The image is a computer-generated representation of a student's hand-drawn and colored VTN, using shapes in place of the student's original color coding. Special thanks to Dr. Mohammed Dalibih, University of Arizona, for his assistance in the creation of this work.

to build a web of relationships. The ideas are represented on paper in the shapes, colors, configurations, and links that depict the student's thinking process. The product is a concrete personal representation of their understanding of the topic (see Figure 11.1).

VTN Procedure

Approval for the pilot project was given by the university institutional review board. Two groups of students were selected from a foundational nursing course to participate in this pilot project. One group received teaching with the VTN strategy; the other group used a narrative activity. After explaining the pilot project and obtaining informed consent, students participated in the traditional asepsis teaching done by course faculty. This content on asepsis was taught using a combination of readings, lecture, faculty demonstration, and hands-on practice. Four skills were taught in this asepsis unit: (1) setting up a sterile field, (2) donning sterile gloves, (3) inserting either a male or female urinary catheter, and (4) changing a dry sterile dressing (DSD). The students practiced in the nursing laboratory, then were tested on one of the four skills by return demonstration to faculty.

BOX 11.1 STEPS IN CREATING A VISUAL THINKING NETWORK

This activity centered on the concept of asepsis. Students were given a list of words related to asepsis to use in creating their VTN.

1. Concepts, usually in the form of nouns, are the main focus of the VTN. Nouns are written in some type of a shape. Each concept appears only once in the VTN.
2. Each concept is connected by a verb, adverb, preposition, or linking word that describes how the nouns are related. These linking words are written above a line connecting the concepts. Concepts can be cross-linked with concepts in different parts of the VTN.
3. The VTN is created around a centering point but does not need to be in the center of the paper. The centering point can be any shape or color the student selects. The centering point is a main concept.
4. Main ideas are represented by branches that come off of the centering point. Subbranches are created off of the main branches, and include subconcepts. These are linked by lines.
5. Each line connecting the concepts will have an arrow on the end of it suggesting the relationship between the concepts.
6. Different types of links between concepts can be used to express relationships. Links can be linear or recursive.
7. Color can be used to help encode knowledge into memory.

Steps based on Longo (2007).

The VTN Group

In addition to the traditional instruction just described, eight students in a VTN group met with a faculty member trained in VTN who explained the process of completing a VTN. The VTN-trained faculty member was not associated with the course. These students were given colored pencils and paper, a list of asepsis concepts, and a verbal explanation about how to complete the VTN. Students were also directed to view a 20-minute video on developing a VTN that was available on the course website. Course faculty verified that each student in the VTN group did, in fact, view the video. Students were instructed to complete the VTN at home and to contact the VTN-trained faculty member with any questions. Box 11.1 provides a list of steps for completing a VTN.

The following week, the VTN-trained faculty member returned to the nursing laboratory to meet with the students to answer questions related to the VTN and to collect the completed VTNs.

The Narrative Group

Eight students in a comparison group also met with the VTN-trained faculty member at the conclusion of the asepsis lab. Students in this group were given the same list of asepsis concepts as the VTN group and asked to write a narrative or draw an image using the words provided. Questions were answered and faculty provided contact information for subsequent questions. Students were given this assignment so that they would have a comparable time with the asepsis content and an activity that engaged their brains. The following week, the VTN-trained faculty member met with the students to collect the narratives.

Both Groups

Two weeks after the asepsis lab, all students were tested on skill acquisition using a skills checklist that identified the key steps to performing one of the four required skills. Students randomly selected a skill to demonstrate and were videotaped performing the skill for clinical faculty. All students were encouraged to describe not only what they were doing but to provide a rationale about why they were performing the skill. This think-aloud strategy was designed to elicit not just procedural but more conceptual knowledge and allow the authors to evaluate conceptual understanding of asepsis. Each student was given the same instructions, was tested using the same equipment, in the same room, and had the same length of time to perform the skill.

EVALUATION OF THE VTN STRATEGY

The effectiveness of the VTN strategy was assessed by comparing the outcomes of the VTN group with the outcome of the narrative (control) group. All students were attending school full-time. The mean age of the students was $19.7 \pm .9$ years. All of the students were white, and 14 (88 percent) were female. The skill demonstrations for both groups were videotaped. Verbal data from blinded videotapes were transcribed verbatim by a research assistant (RA) and rechecked against the videotape for accuracy by the RA. Then, the blinded transcripts were analyzed and coded by the investigators responsible for the pilot project individually, and student utterances were coded as either procedural, if they described the task itself, or conceptual, if the student was explaining the rationale for performing the procedure. For example, if a student said: "I am removing my gloves," the statement was coded as procedural. If a student stated: "I am not going to reach over my sterile field to prevent contamination," the statement was coded as conceptual. The investigators then came together to verify the analysis. In cases of discrepancy in coding, both investigators discussed the definitions before deciding on the appropriate coding of a particular data bit.

Both the total number of procedural and conceptual utterances and the percentage of procedural and conceptual utterances (as a percent of all utterances) were entered into the database for each student. A percentage of utterances was also entered, in addition to the total number, due to a different number of steps in each skill and the possibility for uneven numbers of utterances based on differing numbers of steps.

Additionally, the RA watched the blinded videotapes and scored the students on correct demonstration of the skill using a skill checklist. Each student received a total score ranging from 0 percent to 100 percent for correct demonstration of the skill.

RESULTS

The Mann-Whitney U test was used to test group differences because the data were skewed. Table 11.1 displays the results of the analysis. The VTN and control groups did not significantly differ in grade point average (GPA), overall clinical grades, percent of

TABLE 11.1

Comparison of Treatment (VTN) and Control Groups (no VTN) on Major Study Variables

Variable	Mean ± SD or N (%)		*p*
	VTN (n = 8)	Control (n = 8)	
GPA	2.9 ± .27	3.1 ± .43	.61
Overall clinical grade	87 ± 4.2	90 ± 4.0	.87
Number of conceptual utterances	4.2 ± 1.8	1.4 ± .92	.06
Number of procedural utterances	16.1 ± 3.6	17.9 ± 6.8	.89
% of all utterances that are conceptual	20.7 ± 6.9	8.3 ± 5.5	.05*
% accuracy of skill performance	93 ± 9.1	89 ± 9.1	.39
Selected skill			.87
Gloves and setting up field	1 (12.5)	2 (25)	
Dry sterile dressing	4 (50)	3 (37.5)	
Foley insertion	3 (37.5)	3 (37.5)	

*p = .05.
GPA, grade point average, % skill performance out of 100%.

accuracy of skill demonstration, and total number of procedural and conceptual utterances. Chi-square analysis demonstrated that the skills randomly chosen for demonstration by members of each group did not significantly differ as well. However, when comparing the percentage of conceptual utterances (as a percent of all utterances), the students in the VTN group had significantly more conceptual utterances than those in the control group. When looking at the mean number of conceptual utterances in Table 11.1, the students in the VTN group uttered almost three times the number of conceptual utterances when compared to the control group during the asepsis skill demonstration. These preliminary findings suggest that conceptual understanding, as measured by conceptual utterances, was greater in the group that received the VTN intervention. These linkages were made at a higher level of understanding than procedural data and may represent a deeper understanding of the content.

CHALLENGES OF VTN

To participate in this study, both faculty and students assigned to the VTN group were oriented to the principles of creating a VTN via a video purchased through the author of previous studies using this method. The directions were clear, the ideas were novel, and extra time to view was required. Faculty were invested in this project; however, it was difficult to know if students were motivated or how much time was spent viewing the instructions. There were no "extra" incentives to participate other than to be involved in a study. Also, the student's expectation of a nursing laboratory experience currently does not include the use of drawings and coloring; therefore, the investigators had to convey the seriousness of such efforts.

Another challenge with this new method was to find an adequate control group against which to compare the VTN group. Ideally, the control needs to be similar in time on task but different enough to serve as a comparison.

CONCLUSION

The VTN strategy has been posited to increase a student's understanding of scientific concepts by using an innovative strategy to develop linkages in the brains of learners. By creating connections among concepts, students make meaningful linkages between ideas previously learned and new knowledge. In this small pilot project, one finding was particularly striking. Although this was a small sample, the students in the VTN group uttered almost three times as many conceptual statements as the control group during the asepsis skill demonstration. VTN students made these linkages at a higher level of understanding than procedural data and may represent a deeper understanding of the content. These results support the findings of Longo et al. (2002) that higher-order thinking occurred in students who undertook a VTN strategy when learning earth science concepts.

Students in both groups did not significantly differ in percent accuracy of performing the assigned skill. This finding is not surprising, however, because demonstration of a skill can occur by rote with little understanding of the actual reasons for undertaking the skill. When students are assigned a skill, with a checklist to memorize and perform back, they may not develop higher-order linkages between the principles underlying the skill and the actual performance of the skill. The VTN strategy is one method to potentially increase a student's understanding of the principles of surgical asepsis. Although different in structure and process from concept mapping, these findings support the work of Hsu (2007), who demonstrated that students who undertook a concept mapping intervention had improved metacognitive learning.

It is imperative that faculty consider new methods to increase the learning of nursing skills that are foundational to practice. The environments in which nurses practice today are complex and highly technical. Students need to understand the reasons for performing a skill and also must be able to rapidly recall these principles during nursing care. With further research, the VTN strategy might be one way to promote this level of meaningful learning.

References

Craven, R., & Hirnle, C. (2009). *Fundamentals of nursing: Human health and function* (6th ed.). Philadelphia, PA: Lippincott Williams & Wilkins.

Hsu, L. L. (2004). Developing concept maps from problem-based learning scenario discussions. *Journal of Advanced Nursing, 48*(5), 510–518.

Longo, P. J., Anderson, O. R., & Wicht, P. (2002). Visual thinking networking promotes problem solving achievement for 9th grade earth science students. *The Electronic Journal of Science Education, 7,* 1–50. Retrieved from http://wolfweb.unr.edu/homepage/crowther/ejse/ejsev7n1.html

Longo, P. J. (2007, November). *Causal links between color and cognition in Visual Thinking Networks: Closing the gender gap in science achievement.* Poster presented at the International Mind Brain Education Society Meeting. Fort Worth, TX.

Zull, J. (2002). *The art of changing the brain: Enriching the practice of teaching by exploring the biology of learning.* Sterling, VA: Stylus Publishing.

12

The Clinical Portfolio:
A Success Story in Critical Thinking

Amy M. Barrett, MSN, MEd, RN
Cheryl B. Krieg, MSN, RNC-OB
Sharon J. Kinney, MSN, RN, CNE
Elsie Maurer, MSN, RN, NEA-BC
Patricia McKnight, MSN, RN

In the *Forum on the Future of Nursing* report, the Institute of Medicine (IOM) recommended that nursing programs develop and test new approaches to prelicensure clinical education (IOM, 2010). This report also stated that nursing education must provide students opportunities to demonstrate higher-order critical thinking in the practice setting. The question then becomes, how do we teach higher-order critical thinking, especially clinical reasoning?

Critical thinking is defined by the National League for Nursing (NLN, 2010) as "identifying, evaluating, and using evidence to guide decision making by means of logic and reasoning" (p. 34). Critical thinking is the basis for clinical reasoning and necessary for developing a spirit of inquiry. To engage in clinical reasoning, the nurse must be able to use perceptual acuity, that is, the skill of being attentive and involved (Benner, Malloch, & Sheets, 2010). Focusing the students' perceptual acuity to direct their thinking in patient situations is one way that faculty can engage students in higher-order critical thinking. This, however, requires a change in the traditional approach to clinical education.

THE CLINICAL ACTIVITY PORTFOLIO: A SUCCESS STORY IN CRITICAL THINKING

Teaching and evaluating critical thinking and other higher-order thinking in the clinical setting has been a difficult topic for faculty. For years, nurse educators have sought effective ways to teach critical thinking skills. Many strategies have been discussed in the literature, with varying results. This chapter describes the implementation of a new way of clinical teaching that supports the development of critical thinking as used by one practical nursing program.

In June 2010, nursing faculty attended the NLN Immersion in Evidence-Based Nursing Education Conference in Nashville, Tennessee. One of the major themes from the conference was teaching critical thinking and decision making in the clinical setting. Dr. Linda Caputi presented the Caputi Model for Clinical Education© (Caputi, 2010) which uses a Clinical Activity Portfolio© (CAP). Examples of this model were shared and sample tools were provided as templates for attendees to use to create critical thinking learning opportunities in their respective nursing programs. The workshop provided an objective means of teaching and measuring critical thinking in the clinical setting, which was a weak area of the curriculum at the authors' school.

In August 2010, the faculty implemented a CAP in the clinical setting. The program's four student learning outcomes were used to organize the CAP. These outcomes relate to the nurse as provider of care, communicator, manager of care, and member within the discipline of nursing. Each program outcome area contains multiple student behaviors or clinical objectives that the student must meet. For example, within the provider-of-care program outcome area, students must satisfactorily demonstrate the ability to collect objective and subjective data, determine priority problems, implement appropriate nursing interventions, and evaluate interventions and the plan of care. The CAP learning activities directly related to these outcomes and were used to objectively measure a student's competence in the clinical setting. Utilizing several tools provided at the NLN conference, faculty in the Practical Nursing Program developed learning activities that corresponded to each of the program's clinical objectives that tied to the program outcomes. Tying the CAP activities directly to clinical objectives and overall program student learning outcomes demonstrated internal consistency of the curriculum and offered faculty a means to help students develop and objectively evaluate their progress in increasing critical thinking skills. The CAP replaced the weekly clinical evaluation tool previously used to monitor student progress. Student submissions in their clinical portfolios were evaluated at midterm and at the end of the semester.

Clinical portfolio activities were designed to engage student thinking in the following areas: reflection, prioritizing, comparing, analyzing, and applying. Each week, faculty assigned students to two groups: members of one group were assigned traditional patient care while members of the second group were assigned portfolio activities. Students rotated between patient assignments and clinical portfolio activities weekly. By the end of the first semester, all students had the opportunity to spend several clinical days engaged in traditional patient assignments and several clinical days of focused critical thinking portfolio activities.

Students assigned to portfolio activities had the opportunity to work individually or in pairs when collecting data for their clinical activities. They then presented what they learned from their portfolio activities in postconference, so all students could learn to engage in the various kinds of thinking strategies elicited by the portfolio activities.

Some examples of activities included in the clinical portfolio were:

- Creating a patient problem concept map
- Completing a laboratory work profile
- Completing a patient teaching plan
- Reviewing and comparing institutional safety policies
- Completing an SBAR (Situation, Background, Assessment, Recommendation) report

By the end of the first semester, all faculty noted definite changes in the thinking abilities of their students.

RESULTS

Evidence of the students' higher-order thinking abilities were manifested in a number of ways:

- Students were asking higher-level questions regarding lab values, medications, and other patient care issues than they had previously. Staff members in the clinical setting commented positively about the level of inquiry that students were displaying. This was not the case in previous first semesters.
- Students were engaging in critical thinking discussions with each other and with the faculty during clinical and class much earlier than did students in previous classes.
- Students were recognizing that they were able to make the connections between knowledge acquired in the classroom and its application in the clinical setting, stating that they were feeling like a "real nurse."

By the second semester, faculty were witnessing a difference in the quality of care planning and prioritizing of care in the clinical setting. In class, student dialogue during lecture and case study activities were representative of more in-depth thinking.

In addition to these unexpected behaviors, students were demonstrating an increase in critical thinking ability on examinations. Upon beginning the nursing program, all nursing students completed a standardized critical thinking examination to determine their initial critical thinking level. The group score for the 2010 to 2011 critical thinking

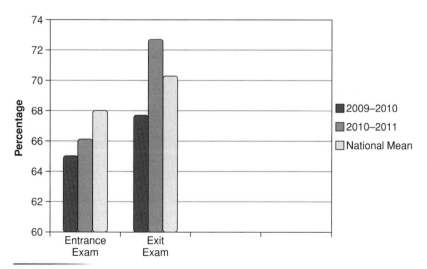

FIGURE 12.1 Student test scores on the critical thinking entrance exam and the critical thinking exit exam, 2009–2010 and 2010–2011.

assessment entrance exam was 66.1%; the national mean score for the exam was 68%. Students were tested again at the end of the second semester to determine if there was a difference in critical thinking ability from the beginning of the year to date. The critical thinking exit exam has traditionally been given in the third semester. The group score for the 2010 to 2011 critical thinking exit exam was 72.7%; the national mean score for the exam was 70.3%. These students scored 2.4 % above the national mean on the critical thinking exit exam.

When comparing beginning and ending test scores from previous classes, it was found that students in the 2010 to 2011 class outscored the previous class by 5 percent. This increase in critical thinking score is attributed to the critical thinking clinical portfolio, as no other program changes had been implemented. Curriculum, textbooks, faculty, and clinical sites remained the same. Figure 12.1 reflects student test scores.

References

Benner, P. E., Malloch, K., & Sheets, V. (Ed.) (2010). *Nursing pathways for patient safety.* St. Louis, MO: Mosby.

Caputi, L. (2010). *Transforming clinical education: The Caputi clinical activities portfolio,* In L. Caputi (Ed.), *Teaching Nursing: The Art and Science, Vol. 2* (2nd ed., pp. 216–255). Glen Ellyn, IL: DuPage Press.

Institute of Medicine (IOM). (2010). *A summary of the February 2010 forum on the future of nursing.* Washington, DC: National Academies Press.

National League for Nursing (NLN). (2010). *Outcomes and competencies for graduates of practical/vocational, diploma, associate degree, baccalaureate, master's, practice doctorate, and research doctorate programs in nursing.* New York, NY: Author.

13

Helping Students with Critical Thinking through Scholarly Writing

Richard L. Pullen, Jr., EdD, RN, CMSRN

Undergraduate nursing students must have scholarly writing experiences that help prepare them for professional practice. Nurses use critical thinking to develop, analyze, and communicate a plan of patient care to the interprofessional team. The nurse's analysis of patient-centered data must be clearly communicated verbally and in writing. Scholarly writing helps students with communication skills by requiring them to use critical thinking that reflects the higher cognitive levels of analysis, synthesis, and evaluation (McMillan & Raines, 2011). Scholarly writing provides students with a foundation to pursue additional nursing education and assume leadership roles in health care organizations, advanced clinical practice (ACP), and academia.

At the Associate Degree Nursing Program at Amarillo Community College, scholarly writing was initially introduced into the associate degree nursing program in 1996 in the critical care clinical setting. Students were required to evaluate patient-centered data to improve nursing practice and present their evaluation in a scholarly paper (Pullen, Reed, & Oslar, 2001). Clinical learning activities, including formal writing, have evolved in the nursing program in response to the National League for Nursing (NLN) mandate to transform clinical education and the emergence of innovative evidence-based models for clinical instruction and evaluation (Caputi, 2010; NLN, 2008; Tanner, 2009; White, 2006). For example, alternate learning activities are included in clinical learning that focus on safety and interprofessional collaboration, and the major care plan has been replaced with formal writing experiences.

The formal writing assignments in the medical-surgical clinical courses among the four levels in the program show progression in the depth and breadth of analysis of patient-centered data:

- Students complete a creative writing assignment in Level One that focuses on the teaching needs of an older adult patient.
- Students prepare a clinical topic paper (CTP) in Level Two that requires them to review the literature on a disease process and then make

recommendations to improve nursing practice. The CTP is a creative writing assignment that also introduces students to some elements of scholarly writing.

- The Level Three clinical synthesis paper (CSP) is the students' first full-emersion experience with scholarly writing. The CSP requires students to analyze and synthesize patient-centered data, evaluate evidence-based literature and its relationship to their patient's clinical status, and develop a plan of patient care from an interprofessional perspective. The CSP comprises 25 percent of the student's clinical grade.

- The CSP establishes a foundational structure for students to be successful in scholarly writing when they prepare the scholarly paper (SP) in the Level Four medical-surgical course (critical care). The CSP and SP are similar in rigor; however, the SP requires more analysis related to the patient's pathophysiology.

THE CLINICAL SYNTHESIS PAPER

Guidelines for the CSP

Guidelines provide students with a detailed step-by-step process for preparing the CSP. Students select a topic of interest from the information that they have organized in a concept map while caring for a patient. The clinical instructor guides the student in the development of the title for the CSP. Examples of titles from previous papers include "Evaluating Mobility in a Patient with Rheumatoid Arthritis" and "Managing Fluid Volume in a Patient with Addison's Disease."

Students prepare a six- to eight-page paper using the American Psychological Association (APA) form and style. Sections of the paper include: (1) Introduction, (2) Patient-Centered Data, (3) Review of Related Literature, (4) Patient-Centered Analysis, (5) Implications for Nursing Practice, and (6) Conclusions. Faculty members team with a college librarian to conduct a three-hour interactive workshop with students on the development of the CSP, including a detailed presentation on the guidelines, grading rubric, APA form and style, database searches, and avoidance of plagiarism. Students then brainstorm topics for the CSP while seated at a computer terminal, guided by faculty members and the librarian as they search for evidence-based citations.

Grading Rubric for the CSP

The grading rubric apprises students of what is expected of them and helps clinical faculty evaluate the CSP consistently and efficiently. In recent years, the inter-rater reliability (IR) has significantly improved through a critical evaluation of the guidelines, grading rubric, and availability of student resources. The grading rubric (Table 13.1) parallels the guidelines. The evaluation key includes a performance number (PN) that corresponds with a level of performance. Each section of the CSP is assigned a percentage. The percentage becomes a conversion factor (CF) that is multiplied by the PN to

TABLE 13.1

Grading Criteria (Rubric) for Clinical Synthesis Paper (Evaluation Key)

PN[a]		Level of Performance
10	Outstanding performance	Complete and organized, and fully and specifically developed.
		Demonstrates depth and breadth in the analysis and synthesis of patient-centered data.
		Demonstrates superior writing ability.
9	Excellent performance	Complete and organized.
		Demonstrates depth and breadth in the analysis and synthesis of patient-centered data.
8	Good performance	Complete and organized.
		Demonstrates many elements of analysis and synthesis of patient-centered data.
7	Satisfactory performance	Generally complete and organized.
		Demonstrates some elements of analysis and synthesis of patient-centered data.
6	Unsatisfactory performance	Not complete and/or organized.
		Demonstrates very little, if any, analysis and synthesis of patient-centered data.
0	Failure	Almost all information lacking and/or student did not address criteria at all.

[a]PN = Performance number × % for each section (CF = conversion factor) = total points

determine the total points for a section. Total points for all sections are multiplied by 10 to determine the final score. For example, total points of 8.7 translate to a grade of 87 percent (see Table 13.2). Table 13.3 presents the APA scoring sheet and Table 13.4 presents the final evaluation of the paper.

OUTCOMES

An evaluation of the CSP as a critical thinking learning tool has been favorable. Since the inception of the CSP in 2004, students have generally performed well on this assignment, with an aggregated mean score of 84.7 percent. Selected comments by students about the CSP on surveys and in clinical rotations include:

- "The paper challenged my critical thinking skills."
- "The paper was difficult to write because I had to keep comparing my patient to the literature."

TABLE 13.2

Clinical Synthesis Paper Scoring Sheet

Criteria	PN × CF	Points
SECTION 1: INTRODUCTION (5 percent)		
1. Provided a brief description of the topic and pathophysiology.	_____ × .05	
2. Briefly discussed why topic is important to nursing practice.		
3. Provided a clearly written purpose statement.		
SECTION 2: PATIENT-CENTERED DATA (10 percent)		
1. Provided sufficient data that supports the topic of paper. Included a discussion of patient-related objective data related to physical, psychological, and spiritual distress. Data includes—but is not limited to—medications, treatments and therapies, diagnostic procedures, imaging studies, laboratory values, and progress notes from the interprofessional team members.	_____ × 0.1	
2. Provided subjective data from the patient, the patient's family, and interprofessional team members.		
SECTION 3: REVIEW OF RELATED LITERATURE (20 percent)		
1. Provided a clearly written introductory paragraph that discusses how the review of literature was conducted.	_____ × .05	
2. Provided 3 clearly written paraphrased citations from evidence-based literature. Identified the main points or themes from each citation.	_____ × 0.1	
3. Provided a clearly written compare and contrast of the author(s) views among the 3 citations.	_____ × .05	
SECTION 4: PATIENT-CENTERED ANALYSIS (30 percent)		
1. Provided a clearly written analysis that shows critical thinking and clinical reasoning of how the patient's clinical status compares with the main points or themes that are presented by the author(s) in each citation.	_____ × 0.1	
2. Provided a clearly written analysis that shows critical thinking and clinical reasoning of how the patient's clinical status contrasts with the main points or themes that are presented by the author(s) in each citation.	_____ × 0.1	
3. Provided an explanation of how the evidence and the patient's clinical status support the need for patient teaching. Clearly presented priority teaching that was identified by the student and patient together.	_____ × 0.1	

TABLE 13.2

Clinical Synthesis Paper Scoring Sheet (*Continued*)

Criteria	PN × CF	Points
SECTION 5: IMPLICATIONS FOR NURSING PRACTICE (30 percent)		
1. Clearly identified one patient-centered safety problem while providing care. Formulated a plan for the nursing profession that will improve this problem. Provided sufficient details showing synthesis (putting the pieces together).	____× 0.15	
2. Created an "ideal" interprofessional team for the patient. Clearly presented what professions would be represented on the team and why. Described why it is important for nurses to be an active voice in interprofessional teamwork.	____× 0.15	
SECTION 6: CONCLUSIONS (5 percent)		
1. Student clearly explained how the care of the patient impacted the student.	____× .05	
2. Described significant learning and how this learning will help prepare the student for nursing practice.		
INSTRUCTOR EVALUATIVE COMMENTS ON SECTIONS 1–6:		

- "Each section of the paper required me to think critically, unlike the major care plan."
- "The CSP and alternate learning activities will help me in the real world of nursing."
- "The paper will help me when I get my BSN."

Employers consistently indicate on annual surveys that critical thinking, clinical reasoning, and communication are among the strengths of our program alumni.

TABLE 13.3

American Psychological Association (APA) Scoring Sheet (Form and Style Evaluation)

Format Topic	Point Deduction (each error)	Instructor Comments
APA title page errors	1	
APA format errors in text	1	
APA grammatical errors	1	
APA punctuation errors	1	
APA reference errors	2	
Spelling errors	2	
Paper length: 6–8 pages of text	1 each line (short or long)	
Paper late	10 each day	
2 copies paper not submitted	5	
Grade sheet not submitted	5	

TABLE 13.4

Final Evaluation of Paper

Section of Paper	Points Earned
Total points Sections 1–6	_____ × 10 = _____
Total points deduction form and style	
Final grade for paper	

_____
Clinical Instructor Signature and Date

References

Caputi, L. (2010). Evaluating students in the clinical setting. In L. Caputi (Ed.), *Teaching Nursing: The Art and Science* (2nd ed.). Glen Ellyn, IL: College of DuPage Press.

McMillan, L. R., & Raines, K. (2011). Using the "write" resources: Nursing student evaluation of an interdisciplinary collaboration using a professional writing assignment. *Journal of Nursing Education, 50*(12), 697–702.

National League for Nursing (NLN). (2008). Transforming clinical nursing education. Retrieved from www.nln.org/faculty-programs/pdf/think_tank.

Pullen, R. L., Reed, K. E., & Oslar, K. (2001). Promoting clinical scholarship through scholarly writing. *Nurse Educator, 26*(2), 81–83.

Tanner, C. (2010). From mother duck to mother lode: Clinical education for deep learning. *Journal of Nursing Education, 49*(1), 3–4.

White, L. L. (2006). Preparing for clinical: Just in time. *Nurse Educator, 31*(2), 57–60.

14

Out of the SimLab and into the Classroom:
Using High-Fidelity Simulation as an Active Classroom Teaching Strategy

Heidi M. Meyer, MSN, RN, PHN

Active teach/learn strategies are critical in teaching nursing students. The call for radical transformation in nursing education by the Carnegie Foundation for the Advancement of Teaching emphasizes the need for active engagement of students in the classroom (Benner, Sutphen, Leonard, & Day, 2010). "Classroom teachers must step out from behind their screen full of slides and engage students in clinic-like learning experiences that ask them to learn to use knowledge and practice thinking in changing situations, always for the good of the patients" (Benner et al., 2010, p. 14). *Teaching Nursing: The Art and Science* also stresses the need for active learning strategies in the classroom (Caputi, 2010). "Although lecture is a popular method for delivering instruction in the classroom, lecture should be enhanced or replaced with active learning strategies that require the students to engage in critical thinking" (Caputi, 2010, p. 421). This chapter describes how high-fidelity simulation (HFS) was used during classroom theory as an active teach/learn strategy.

BACKGROUND

Experiential learning pedagogies and problem-based learning (PBL) constructs are found throughout nursing literature (Parker & Myrick, 2010; Ravert, 2008; Walshe, O'Brien, Murphy, & Hartigan, 2013). Simulation as an active teach/learn strategy reinforces these pedagogies in nursing curricula and creates an environment that fosters critical thinking and clinical reasoning. "Building on didactic content, the active, experiential learning experiences of simulation reinforce concepts and take the student from the level of basic knowledge to application and synthesis" (Durham & Alden, 2010, p. 35). Studies of the use of HFS as an experiential learning method for teaching are increasingly seen in the nursing literature. However, the majority of research on simulation focuses on the benefits of simulation used with small groups of students in a clinical scenario as a way to teach concepts applicable in practice (Brewer, 2011).

With the majority of simulation research spotlighting small groups with a clinical focus, little research exists on the effects of using HFS during a didactic course. In a study by Brannan, White, & Bezanson (2008), junior-level baccalaureate nursing students were instructed on the care of an acute myocardial infarction patient. These students were divided into two groups: one group received the traditional lecture method while the other received instruction using a human patient simulator (HPS). Comparing pre- and posttest acute myocardial infarction questionnaire results, students who received the instruction with the HPS achieved significantly higher posttest scores than did students who received the traditional lecture approach (Brannan, White, & Bezanson, 2008). In another study, an HPS was used as a teaching strategy in a classroom of 45 associate degree nursing students (Beyer, 2011). The results of pre- and posttests showed significant learning occurred and students positively rated the classroom simulation. Beyer (2011) concludes that simulation activities may be used in larger groups as an interactive and engaging teaching strategy (p. e1).

USING SIMULATION IN THE CLASSROOM

A simulation day was implemented with 26 junior-level bachelor of nursing students during their class on congestive heart failure (CHF). A simulation scenario of a patient in heart failure was used to meet the class objectives for the day. The scenario was broken into four parts for faculty organization. The scenario took approximately 60 minutes to run.

Preparation

Students prepared for the day by reviewing learning objectives and assigned readings found in the course manual. The HFS was prepped with the CHF scenario. A faculty member dressed as the wife of the 67-year-old simulated patient, donning a gray-haired wig and spectacles. After approximately 5 minutes of students waiting for class to start, the faculty member entered the classroom, pushing the simulated patient in with a wheelchair.

Part I: Introduction

The faculty member role-played the wife of the simulated patient throughout the scenario, framing questions to students as if the students were nurses (in first-person and present tense format). The scenario was introduced to students upon initial entrance to the classroom via questioning students about events in the emergency department (ED). An assessment/documentation form was brought in and given to one student, asking to have the events documented. All students were encouraged to take notes as the scenario progressed.

Part 2: Assessment

The HFS was left at the front of the classroom, while the patient's wife (the faculty member) walked around, engaging individual students and asking direct questions. The questioning about CHF began with a focus on pathophysiology and the disease process. More questions were asked about risk factors. These questions prompted students to ask direct health history questions that contribute to CHF. Students were then asked if there was anything else they would like to know about the patient. More questions ensued related to physiology, specifically medications used, as well as psychosocial and sociocultural variables. During the question session, it became evident that the "wife" was a little forgetful.

Physical assessment of the patient came next. Continuing to play the wife, the faculty member asked students to approach the HFS and assess specific areas related to CHF exacerbation. Students assessed lung sounds, oxygen saturation, heart rate, and heart sounds, and asked about current weight. A peripheral assessment, which included checking pedal pulses and edema, was also completed. Students were asked why they were assessing specific areas. For example, while students were checking for pedal edema, they were asked the causes of edema. Other questions were asked about specific concepts that faculty wanted to ensure were understood. Throughout the questioning, the environment was supportive and collaborative. With the data gathered, students were prompted to notify the health care provider. The documenter called the provider and stated the significant assessment findings in Situation Background Assessment Response (SBAR) format.

Part 3: The Orders

The students were given orders to implement with the patient. The orders were placed on an overhead projector for analysis. Orders included activity restrictions, diet, weight, intake and output monitoring, labs to be drawn, oxygen and medications to be administered, and diagnostic tests to be completed. The faculty member continued to role-play the patient's wife and asked individual students questions related to every order given. For example, when the diuretic was discussed, pharmacodynamics was discussed as well as specific nursing assessments that needed to occur to monitor for effects and side effects of this medication. Students were validated or corrected, all while still in the role-play. After all orders were reviewed, the patient was ready to be admitted and the scenario ended.

Part 4: Debriefing

After a brief break, students debriefed. Small breakout groups were used for the first 15 minutes to review data and to create two to three nursing diagnoses with interventions. After small group work, students were brought together to collaborate as a class to create a large concept map on the board. Data on the concept map included pathophysiology, risk factors, lab/diagnostic tests, medications, and assessment data that supported the multiple nursing diagnoses chosen. Faculty reviewed evidence-based nursing

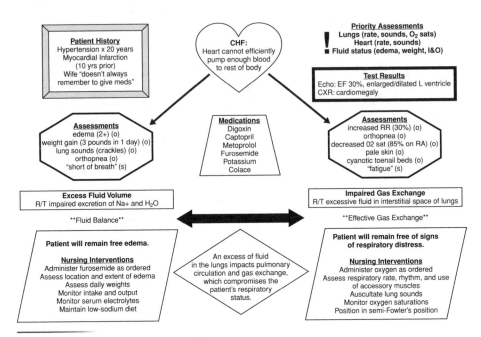

FIGURE 14.1 Sample Concept Map

interventions and rationale as well as reinforced specific concepts related to overall class objectives. The concept map debriefing took approximately 50 minutes. Figure 14.1 provides an example of the concept map.

CONCLUSION AND FUTURE DIRECTION

The active teach/learn strategy of implementing HFS into classroom theory was used to teach principles of CHF exacerbation. Implementing HFS into theory content reinforced the importance of creating a learning environment that encourages students' active participation, as well as cooperation and collaboration with their peers. Students were notably engaged and eager to participate. On overall evaluations from students exposed to HFS in the classroom, 96 percent agreed that this faculty member provided a stimulating atmosphere for learning and critical thinking. Comments from students included:

- "Stimulates critical thinking."
- "Wants us to think critically and engage to learn about the material."
- "Stimulates the students to think about the BIG picture."
- "Stimulates us to think deeper and make connections."

With the majority of literature spotlighting small student groups with a clinical focus, more research needs to occur on the effects of using HFS as an interactive teach/learn approach in a classroom setting. Future research should include comparisons of learning outcomes using HFS scenarios versus traditional lecture or other interactive teach/learn strategies.

References

Benner, P., Sutphen, M., Leonard, V., & Day, L. (2010). *Educating nurses: A call for radical transformation*. San Francisco, CA: Jossey-Bass.

Beyer, D. A. (2011). Effectiveness of human patient simulator as a classroom teaching strategy. *Clinical Simulation in Nursing*. e1–e5. doi: 10.1016/j.ecns.2011.01.005.

Brannan, J. D., White, A., & Bezanson, J. L. (2008). Simulator effects on cognitive skills and confidence levels. *Journal of Nursing Education, 47*(11), 495–500.

Brewer, E. P. (2011). Successful techniques for using human patient simulation in nursing education. *Journal of Nursing Scholarship, 43*(3), 311–317. doi: 10.1111/j.1547-5069.2011.01405.x

Caputi, L. (2010). Ideas to develop critical thinking in the classroom and clinical setting. In L. Caputi (Ed.), *Teaching nursing: The art and science, Vol. 2* (2nd ed., pp. 413–431). Glen Ellyn, IL: College of DuPage Press.

Durham, C. F., & Alden, K. R. (2010). The nuts and bolts of using simulation. In L. Caputi (Ed.), *Teaching nursing: The art and science, Vol. 2* (2nd ed., pp. 28–55). Glen Ellyn, IL: College of DuPage Press.

Parker, B., & Myrick, F. (2010). Transformative learning as context for human patient simulation. *Journal of Nursing Education, 49*(3), 1–8.

Ravert, P. (2008). Patient simulator sessions and critical thinking. *Journal of Nursing Education, 47*(12), 557–562.

Walshe, N., O'Brien, S., Murphy, S., & Hartigan, I. (2013). Integrative learning through simulation and problem-based learning. *Clinical Simulation in Nursing* (article in press). 9(2), e1–e8.

15

Mid-Scenario Reflection:
A Teaching Strategy for Simulation in Nursing Education

Kimberly H. Raines, PhD, CRNP

The use of high-fidelity simulation (HFS) is relatively new in nursing education, though its use is growing (Katz, Peifer, & Armstrong, 2010; Nehring & Lashley, 2004). However, there is a dearth of knowledge regarding best HFS practices (Kardong-Edgren, Adamson, & Fitzgerald, 2010; Prion, 2008) and the current literature lacks specific recommendations regarding the role of the facilitator in simulation (Jeffries, 2005). This chapter describes the use of an innovative HFS teaching strategy: mid-scenario reflection.

Mid-scenario reflection is defined by this author as a brief hiatus during a simulation exercise in which student-participants engage in an instructor-guided reflective discussion period. This "time out" provides students an opportunity to consider the gathered patient assessment information and develop a plan for nursing care that is then implemented once the scenario resumes. This teaching technique has been neither studied nor described in the literature.

THE OBSTETRICAL SIMULATION DESIGN

The mid-scenario reflection teaching strategy was implemented at a school of nursing offering a baccalaureate nursing degree and located in a public university in the southeastern United States. In the junior year, students enroll in a women's health course that offers didactic and clinical instruction in obstetrical and gynecological nursing. Part of the 90-hour clinical component includes an HFS with the manikin, Noelle®. Noelle is manufactured by Gaumard Scientific® and is a high-fidelity reproduction of an average-sized adult. The manikin is equipped with an interactive software package that allows the operator to reproduce normal and abnormal physiologic conditions encountered in practice; its features include the ability to simulate labor and birth.

The simulation laboratory consists of two large rooms that replicate an inpatient clinical setting. One room contains the low-fidelity manikins and task trainers. The room that houses Noelle contains two other HFS manikins as well. Noelle is situated on an electronically controlled hospital bed in a realistic representation of an inpatient labor room. Noelle is connected to monitors that display vital signs—temperature, pulse, respiration, and oxygen saturation—in addition to a fetal monitor that displays real-time contractions and the fetal heart rate.

The "hospital room" also features a bedside table with simulated oxygen and suction equipment situated on a wall panel. The room is equipped with a telephone, clock, and bedside computer that displays Noelle's medical record. Microphones and cameras are at the bedside of each HFS manikin. A control booth installed behind a one-way glass window contains the computer controls for the manikins and an audio system allows communication between simulation participants and operators/faculty inside the booth.

Students enrolled in the women's health course are expected to complete an HFS experience as part of the clinical requirement. Students were scheduled for an HFS session offered on eight different days over a four-week period with two groups scheduled per day. Each group consists of three randomly assigned students, who are given 35 minutes in which to complete the obstetrical scenario.

Prior to the HFS, the students received classroom content on the pathophysiology and nursing care of a full-term pregnant patient with chorioamnionitis. Students prepared further for the experience by reading the written HFS objectives (Box 15.1) prior to the simulation.

A term pregnancy chorioamnionitis scenario was developed by faculty for use in this study. The chorioamnionitis condition was chosen because students are seldom able to care for such patients due to the high-risk nature of the complication. The physiological events involved in chorioamnionitis were programmed into the simulator by faculty. Communication by the patient included such statements as "I feel terrible," "I've never hurt so bad in my life," and "I'm burning up." The fetal heart rate was programmed at the elevated rate of 158 to 168 beats per minute with moderate variability. Noelle's vital sign monitor displayed a temperature of 101.4°F with an elevated heart rate of 102 and elevated respiratory rate of 22. Once the appropriate interventions were accomplished, the fetal heart rate, maternal heart rate, respiratory rate, and temperature returned to normal levels. Table 15.1 illustrates the outline for the scenario.

BOX 15.1 SIMULATION OBJECTIVES OF THE OBSTETRICAL SCENARIO

At the conclusion of the scenario, the student will be able to:

1. Perform basic nursing skills necessary in giving care to the laboring patient
2. Assess uterine contractions, including intensity, duration, and frequency
3. Assess fetal well-being during labor
4. Analyze the laboring patient's reaction to drugs received during the labor process
5. Develop a plan of care for the laboring patient experiencing complications using the nursing process
6. Communicate effectively with the health care team

TABLE 15.1

Scenario Outline of High-Fidelity Simulation of Term Pregnancy Chorioamnionitis

Time Frame	Patient Responses	Expected Student Performance	Patient Cues
Assessment (5–10 min)	T: 101.4°F P: 102 R: 22 FHR: 166 Lung sounds: Clear Cervix: 5/80%/0 station Contractions: 3–5 min for 60 sec with moderate intensity	Introduce self. Perform hand hygiene. Conduct initial assessment. Recognize abnormal findings. Discuss patient's status and the need to call the CNM.	"I've never hurt so bad in my life." "I'm burning up." "Please get me something for this pain." "Is my baby OK?"
Reflection/ Planning (5 min)		Discuss patient assessment, plan, interventions, and expected outcomes	
Intervention (10 min)	T: 101.5°F P: 104 R: 22 FHR: 142 Contractions: 3–5 min for 60 sec with moderate intensity	Call CNM. Explain rationales for medications. Verify allergies. Administer IV antibiotic, pain medication, acetaminophen. Instruct patient regarding relaxation techniques.	"I'm not allergic to anything." "How long will this pain medicine take to work?"
Reevaluation (10 min)	T: 99.5°F P: 84 R: 16 FHR: 142 Contractions: 3–5 min for 60 sec with moderate intensity	Continue to monitor patient, fetal status, and labor progression. Document care.	"I'm starting to feel better."

CNM, Certified Nurse Midwife; FHR, fetal heart rate; P, pulse; R, respiratory rate; T, temperature.

Immediately before participating in the HFS, students were informed about the schedule of events for the simulation; the written objectives for the exercise were then reviewed. Students next received a brief orientation to the manikin and the simulation laboratory. Participants were randomly assigned to a role for the simulation—roles included that of primary nurse, secondary nurse, and nurse-recorder. The primary nurse was responsible for leading the team in patient care, although all students were expected to be involved directly in the patient's care.

Two instructors were placed in the laboratory control booth—one operated the manikin and spoke for both the patient and the Certified Nurse Midwife (CNM) while the other observed the students. There was no instructor at the bedside.

One instructor played the role of the reporting nurse. Students received a verbal report from the nurse/instructor who cared for the patient since admission and were given an opportunity to ask questions of the nurse. The students then entered the patient's room and the instructor entered the control booth. The students interacted with the patient, obtained initial physical assessment data, and discussed the findings as a group. Students held a discussion regarding the patient's abnormal assessment findings and invariably reached a decision to call the CNM.

Once the students reached the point when it became necessary to telephone the CNM to provide an update regarding the patient's status and to receive new medication and treatment orders, the instructor stopped the simulation. The group then adjourned to an adjacent classroom for a 5- to 10-minute, instructor-led, guided reflection period that included a discussion regarding assessment findings and the nursing diagnoses based on the findings. The group mutually developed a plan of care, then returned to the simulation lab to resume the scenario and implement planned interventions.

The nursing process was used as a framework for the mid-scenario discussion. The nursing process consists of assessment, problem identification, intervention, planning, and implementation (American Nurses Association [ANA], 2004). Use of the nursing process was an attempt on the part of the instructor to guide clinical reasoning in a structured manner using an existing cognitive framework with which the students were already familiar.

The scenario ended when students administered intravenous (IV) pain medication, an IV antibiotic, and an oral dose of acetaminophen or when 35 minutes had elapsed, whichever came first. Following the conclusion of the scenario, the students participated in a 15- to 20-minute postsimulation debriefing. Student feelings, opinions, and responses during the scenario were discussed.

FACULTY EVALUATION OF THE MID-SCENARIO REFLECTION DESIGN

Faculty participants and faculty observers noted that the obstetrical scenario provided students the opportunity to solve problems, apply clinical judgment, and practice psychomotor skills. Students also practiced communication skills with the patient, team members, and the CNM. The inclusion of the mid-scenario reflective period also provided an opportunity to experience reflection in action, an important thinking skill nurses use.

Each student group successfully cared for the patient within the allotted time. In past simulation experiences when no mid-scenario reflection took place, students appeared dissatisfied with their performance. Students often stated: "It all happened so fast" and "I wish there was more time to think about what the patient needed." In contrast, with the mid-scenario reflection, students regarded their performance more positively. The students valued the opportunity to experience a pause in the action to reflect. Several students stated that they felt confident about caring for an actual patient with chorioamnionitis as a result of the simulation experience.

Students made many anecdotal comments specific to the mid-scenario reflection. Several noted: "I felt more confident about talking to the nurse-midwife because I knew what my plan of care should be and exactly what I wanted to communicate." Several students also stated: "Taking the time-out gave me a chance to think about what I needed to do for the patient." Another frequent comment was: "This experience gives me more confidence to go into a real clinical situation."

CONCLUSIONS

One distinct advantage of using the mid-scenario reflection design is that only two instructors were needed to facilitate the simulation. Prior to using the mid-scenario strategy, three instructors were needed: one spoke for the patient, one played the role of the reporting nurse and the CNM, and one was at the bedside to assist students.

Although faculty were satisfied with the incorporation of the mid-scenario reflection for this group of students, this method may not be successful with other simulation participants. For example, experienced simulation participants, such as highly-skilled RNs, might consider the mid-scenario pause to be a distracting interruption.

The incorporation of a mid-scenario reflection period was a successful teaching strategy for this group of junior-level baccalaureate students participating in a high-fidelity obstetrical simulation. However, quantitative studies are warranted to examine whether this is an effective teaching strategy. A study is underway by this author to explore the impact of the mid-scenario reflection on learning outcomes.

Using simulations, nurse educators create patient care situations to meet program learning outcomes in a controlled environment without risk to the patient. Although the use of an HFS in nursing education is increasing, there is a paucity of evidence regarding best teaching strategies for optimizing learning outcomes (Jeffries, 2005; Kardong-Edgren, Adamson, & Fitzgerald, 2010; Prion, 2008). More research is needed as nurse educators use the simulation literature to determine best practices for simulation use in nursing education programs (Harder, 2009). This initial experience in incorporating a mid-scenario reflection into an HFS appears to be an effective teaching strategy.

References

American Nurses Association (ANA). (2004). *Nursing: Scope and standards of practice.* Washington, DC: Author.

Harder, N. (2009). Evolution of simulation use in health care education. *Clinical Simulation in Nursing, 5,* 169–172. doi: 10.1016/j.ecns.2009.04.092

Jeffries, P. (2005). A framework for designing, implementing, and evaluating simulations used as teaching strategies in nursing.

Nursing Education Perspectives, 26(2), 96–103.

Kardong-Edgren, S., Adamson, K., & Fitzgerald, C. (2010). A review of currently published evaluation instruments for human patient simulation. *Clinical Simulation in Nursing, 6,* 25–35. doi: 10.1016/j.ecns.2009.08.004

Katz, G., Peifer, K., & Armstrong, G. (2010). Assessment of patient simulation use in selected baccalaureate nursing programs in the United States. *Simulation in Healthcare, 5*(1), 46–51.

Nehring, W., & Lashley, F. (2004). Current use and opinions regarding human patient simulators in nursing education: An international survey. *Nursing Education Perspectives, 25*(5), 244–248.

Prion, S. (2008). A practical framework for evaluating the impact of clinical simulation experiences in prelicensure nursing education. *Clinical Simulation in Nursing, 4*(3), e69–e78. doi: 10.1016/j.ecns.2008.08.002

16

"We're There to Care for Them as a Whole": Art and Reflection in Clinical Nursing Experience

Carrie A. Bailey, MSN, RN, ACNS-BC
C. Amelia Davis, PhD

[Art] is a reminder to me to take the time to get to know my patients…because they're not just a physical body that needs to be taken care of. They're an emotional body that needs to be taken care of. (Allie)

Finding new ways to encourage nursing students to think holistically about patient care can be a challenge for nursing educators. Many clinical nursing instructors are continually trying to design creative activities for their students that will provide them with the best clinical experiences possible (Bevis, 1988; Casey, 2009). Nursing instructors often look to other disciplines to enhance their teaching practice and foster critical thinking, which "involves evaluating one's own thinking, reflecting on one's actions, and being creative" (Valiga & Bruderle, 1997, p. 7). According to Smith et al. (2004), the integration of the humanities in nursing education "reinforces the balance between the art and science of nursing" (p. 278). In an effort to design an engaging curriculum for clinical nursing education and recognizing that nursing students can become easily overwhelmed with the technical aspect of nursing, we wanted to provide clinical nursing students the opportunity to think reflexively about their work and their position as nurses in relation to that of the care of patients and their families. We wanted to encourage the students to participate actively as learners, share their clinical experiences, and discuss new ways to find meaning in the human experience. We also sought to explore how the use of art could broaden nursing students' perceptions of holistic care and help them better understand comprehensive patient care. Thus, we turned to the humanities, weaving art into our clinical curriculum.

ART AND NURSING EDUCATION

The humanities is "a branch of knowledge that deals with what it means to be human, to live authentically, and share with others" (Valiga & Bruderle, 1997, p. 11). Humanities have been widely integrated into nursing practice in various ways. Carper (1978) stated that

119

there are four fundamental patterns of knowing related to nursing: empirics/science of nursing, esthetic/art of nursing, personal, and ethics/moral knowledge of nursing (p. 14). The esthetic pattern of knowing in nursing involves "the perception of abstracted particulars as distinguished from the recognition of abstracted universals...It is the knowing of a unique particular rather than an exemplary class" (p. 18). The esthetic pattern of knowing in nursing involves the going beyond mere recognition by actively gathering details and scattered particulars into an "experienced whole for the purpose of seeing what is there" (p. 17). The challenge for nurse educators becomes how to develop or reinforce this esthetic pattern of knowing in nurses.

In the years since Carper's article, various health educators have turned to art, the presence of which in hospitals traces back to the 14th century, as a pathway to achieving this esthetic pattern of knowing in individuals (Staricoff, 2006). Why art? Because art is "the expression or application of creative skill and imagination," which produces works that involve individual perception to see the whole of what is there, which often invoke feelings and emotion in individuals, and that give us insight into the human condition (Art, 2010). Ponto (2003) notes that visual art experiences have been incorporated into some health sciences programs and have been used in various ways. Art has been used as a means of allowing students to express their personal philosophy of nursing by utilizing their own artistic skills (Whitman, 2003). Inskeep and Lisko (2001) accompanied a group of clinical nursing students to an art museum and asked them to view certain pictures as they would a patient or their family. Based on their observations, the students were asked to make diagnoses of the individual or family given the defining characteristic they saw. The students described "the experience as a challenging, creative way to make them develop and refine their ability to formulate nursing diagnoses and promote their critical-thinking skills" (Inskeep & Lisko, 2001, p. 119). Some stated that the experience helped them look beyond what was easily seen in the picture, something they felt would "help them look at the total patient situation in the future" (p. 119).

Although Inskeep's and Lisko's work was anecdotal, a more recent study using two groups of nursing students provides us with more empirical evidence of incorporating art into the nursing curriculum. In Pellico's (2009) study, one group of nursing students received traditional classroom and clinical learning instruction. Another group participated in a program using museum artwork that focused on "visual experiences to learn to discriminate, compare, and contrast artistic intentions, as well as learn how to decode objects' meanings and extract information by direct observation" (p. 650). All students in the study were provided six patient photographs to view and record observations in writing. The group that had participated in the program using museum artwork made significantly more written observations and noted more clinical factors associated with emphysema than the traditionally instructed group (p. 651). These studies support the notion that incorporating art in nursing education can be used to supplement traditional teaching methods to improve students' nursing skills, and the inclusion of art does not mean that traditional methods of instruction should be discontinued. Another recent study suggests further benefits for using art as a means for developing the art of nursing. Jensen and Curtis (2008) used art, literature, music, and film in a nursing class as a way to "enhance critical thinking skills and develop empathy in students" (p. 1). As these studies have demonstrated, including art prior to clinical experiences can have substantial merit; however, art can be used in postclinical experiences as a way of facilitating further learning. Art can provide a mechanism for encouraging self-reflection, thereby bringing about a better understanding of self and the patient.

THE STUDY: USING ARTS-BASED EDUCATION TO SUPPORT COMPREHENSIVE PATIENT CARE

Study Background

Although literature supports the integration of art into nursing education, little research is available to support integration of art into the postclinical experience. This research is focused and framed specifically on clinical nursing students and the integration of art into the clinical curriculum. In this exploratory qualitative study, we considered how the use of art in the postclinical nursing experience could broaden nursing students' perceptions of holistic care by engaging in reflective practice and utilizing arts-based resources to increase awareness of comprehensive patient care.

The following research question guided this study: What is the impact of arts-based instruction on nursing students' perceptions of their own nursing practice?

Conceptual Framework

Our conceptual framework informed our participant sample, data collection, data analysis, and interpretation. Methodology for this study is informed by the tenets of arts-based education research (Barone & Eisner, 1997) and Rose's (2001) critical visual methodology to "enhance perspectives" of clinical nursing education (Barone & Eisner, 1997, p. 96). We use a constructivist epistemology, the belief that knowledge is socially constructed (Hatch, 2002), and work within a constructivist research paradigm that presumes multiple realities exist and are constructed by individual experiences (Grbich, 2007).

Arts-based education research (ABER), introduced by Barone and Eisner (1997), reminds us that we have the ability to make sense of the world around us in multiple ways. At times, the meaning of our experiences escapes verbal description and is best represented through visual or structural images. Because images invite us to speak about experiences with reflective depth, for this research, we have chosen to employ ABER not through a linguistic medium but through visual imagery. The structural framework of ABER uses the following seven tenets: (1) the creation of a virtual reality, (2) the presence of ambiguity, (3) the use of expressive language, (4) the use of contextualized and vernacular language, (5) the promotion of empathy, (6) the personal signature of the researcher/writer, and (7) the presence of aesthetic form (Barone & Eisner, 1997). Of these, we consider *the creation of virtual reality, the presence of ambiguity,* and *the promotion of empathy* paramount to our study. *The creation of a virtual reality* is constructed to illustrate physical realities easily recognizable that allow the examiner to identify similarities between the art and personal experience. Through art, students can create their own *virtual reality* as they draw connections and identify similarities between what is depicted in the art and their reality with a patient. The *presence of ambiguity* reminds us that rather than being final statements on what is reality, the research is intentionally open-ended. By encouraging students to engage with artwork, they are invited to make personal meaning from their own experience yet acknowledge the multiple interpretations that are possible. *The promotion of empathy* allows the student to feel the emotions or thoughts of the patient. Such empathic understanding is made possible using evocative artwork that draws the student in to feel as if he or she or the patient is portrayed in the image.

In addition to ABER, we also turned to Rose's (2001) critical visual methodology. In Rose's work the visual is presented as being central to our underestimating and interpretation of the world; we see before we can speak, and we interact with the world largely by seeing it (Hall, 1997). Addressing the need for more rigorous analytical frameworks for arts-based research, particularly as it relates to visual methodologies and data, Rose suggests three critical elements in her approach to critical visual methodology: (1) take images seriously rather than as a pleasant distraction or a reflection of their social contexts; (2) consider the effects of the images and the social conditions in which they were interpreted; (3) practice reflexivity when examining and interpreting images, recognizing that our own social, cultural, political, and historical experiences are tightly coupled with (Weick, 1976) our examination and interpretation of images. We used Rose's methodology to frame our work and our interpretations because it supports the critical reflection we advocate in our own practice and our position that reflexivity aids in understanding that our interpretations are fluid and only momentarily fixed in a particular time and space.

Research Participants

Participants were chosen through convenience sampling (Miles & Huberman, 1994). Junior-year nursing students currently enrolled in a clinical nursing course focused on medical-surgical nursing were asked to participate. There were eight white female participants who were 20 or 21 years of age, all working toward a bachelor of science degree in nursing. These students were asked to participate since they had completed one year of coursework in a baccalaureate nursing program and had just finished a six-week clinical in the hospital setting. Institutional review board approval was obtained before asking students to participate. We, as researchers, were aware of possible ethical implications because the students could have felt compelled to participate in the project because the primary researcher was their clinical instructor. This was discussed with the students and they were assured that there would be no negative repercussions if they chose not to participate in the project. Participation was voluntary and informed consent was obtained. Discussion of the students' representations of their clinical experiences through art was consensual (Casey, 2009).

Research Design

We employed a constructivist research design (Creswell, 2007) that utilized ethnographic methods including participant observation and interviews (Grbich, 2007; Hammersly & Atkinson, 1994). As qualitative researchers we recognize the importance of our own position within our research. We considered our own assumptions about this project and hopes for the broader group of nursing educators by reflecting on our own position including a priori theory, personal philosophy of education, experience in the field, and relationship to the participants (Noblit, Flores, & Murillo, 2004; Pillow, 2003). In this research, we had firsthand knowledge of the students through our positions as instructor and participant observer, respectively, inquiring into their experiences and collecting their narratives and creative interpretations. All the data we draw upon in re-presenting the experiences of the students is drawn from what they shared with us. We acknowledge that interpretations are always partial and positional. The lens through which we interpret our students' words is laced with our own experiences and perceptions of nursing and patient care. Through this research we position ourselves as instructors, researchers, fellow students, and potential patients as we unpack the multidimensional layers of life, experience, and emotion reported to us.

Data Collection

Data were collected through direct observation and recording of student presentations on the last day of the nursing students' clinical rotation.[i] A postconference was held off-site at the home of another nursing instructor with a passion for art. Each student was asked to select an image of artwork from one of the many books available. The students were asked to consider the following when choosing their artwork: (1) choose a picture that represented or reminded them of a patient they had recently cared for, or (2) that represented their own feelings toward a patient they had recently cared for. Each student presented the artwork he or she had chosen to the class, explaining why that particular piece of art was chosen. We engaged the students in unstructured dialogue following each oral presentation. Observation notes were written and each presentation was digitally recorded and then transcribed. When the transcriptions were made, all references that might identify the student were removed and the pseudonym the student chose was used.

Data Analysis and Interpretations

Drawing on tenets of ABER (Barone & Eisner, 2006) and critical visual methodology (Rose, 2001), we coded the data looking for elements of the students' ability to draw connections among the art, their reality with a patient, and their ability to critically reflect upon their experience. Open coding followed by in vivo and sociologically constructed coding (Coffey & Atkinson, 1996; Strauss, 1987) were used to identify categories and themes within and across participants' storied experiences (Glesne, 2007). In vivo codes are derived directly from the language used by the participants in the course of interviews. These codes can often lead the researcher toward associated theoretical codes.

---

[i]**Clinical Program Overview**

The clinical experience begins for students in the first semester of their junior year. In their first semester, the clinical component of their coursework includes students spending one day a week for 12 weeks in the hospital setting interacting and caring for patients. The clinical experience of the second semester of their junior year is similar in format except that the students spend two days a week for six weeks working with patients, and students are required to complete two clinical observation periods. The clinical experience is a hands-on learning during which the students work under the close supervision of a clinical nursing instructor. The instructor chooses patients for the students who will require nursing care for the two days that the students are at the hospital. The students are required to submit a plan of care each week based on their assignment. The students are encouraged to include multiple aspects of the patients' care in order to make them think more holistically about their patients. Once assigned a patient, the students work with the nurses on the unit and the instructor to ensure proper delivery of care. The students and patients interact as they normally would in any nurse-patient situation.

Sociologically constructed codes are developed based on the researcher's knowledge of the field of study. These codes go beyond in vivo codes to "broader social science concerns," adding more depth and utility for analysis (Strauss, 1987, pp. 33–34). Our in vivo codes included faith, hope, and holistic care. Sociologically constructed codes included reflection, empathy, prioritization of care, and emotions. Finally, the following categories and subthemes were developed by identifying commonalities across transcripts: (1) holistic care, subthemes being communication and prioritization of care; (2) reflection, subthemes being care, patient, and self; (3) emotions woven throughout reflection, subthemes being faith, hope, empathy, frustration, and regret.

Keeping with the tenor of arts-based research, we used poetic re-presentations[1] as a means of maintaining students' voices in this article. Face validity (Lather, 1986), agreement between the researcher and participant interpretations, was used to add to the credibility of the data and our interpretations of the students' stories. To capture the tone of self-disclosure and experience that were shared and to draw you, the reader, toward the students' stories and experiences, the poems re-presented here were constructed entirely from the words of the students and placed alongside the artwork they chose to represent their experience. The titles of each poem are direct quotes.

FINDINGS

Using ABER to explore clinical students' experiences enabled us, along with the students, to articulate a wide range of perspectives and impressions regarding "our own world of nursing and the worlds of people in our care" (Casey, 2009, p. 73). For the purposes of this paper, we present our re-presentation of data[2] signaling themes that emerged within and across students' experiences. Two major themes, each including their own subthemes, were developed from the data: (1) holistic care, subthemes being communication and prioritization of care and (2) emotion, subthemes being faith, hope, empathy, frustration, and regret. These themes manifest through reflexivity of holistic care and emotion. Following our re-presentation of the data, we will discuss each of these themes in more detail.

Holistic Care

I Am Sure He Has a Story (Louise's Poem)

He had suffered several mini strokes.
He had right-sided weakness.
You could tell his mind was
very deteriorated.
It was a struggle for him just to communicate.
You could tell he had so much to say

---

[1]The data are "re-presented" because they are a product of our interpretation yet have been carefully constructed to allow student voices to be heard, rather than the voice of the researchers.

[2]Not all data re-presentations could be presented in this article. We have selected poems that we feel most effectively portray the theme under which they are listed.

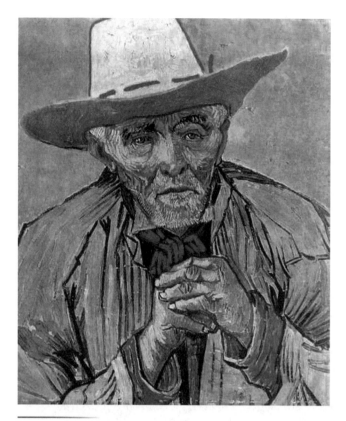

FIGURE 16.1 *Old Peasant* by Vincent Van Gogh (1888).

But
It was like he had someone holding a hand over their mouth.
He just couldn't,
    even though they probably wanted to.
He's probably gotten used to people
    not taking the time to talk to him anymore
So
He just doesn't put forth an effort
    to talk to you that much.
I think I should've tried to talk to him more.
I should have put more of an effort into just talking more to him
    not necessarily trying to get something out of him.
Me give more to him,
    That's what I should've done.
He's probably worked hard his entire life.
He probably doesn't get the credit that he deserves.
I am sure he has a story
But
He can't tell us what it is.

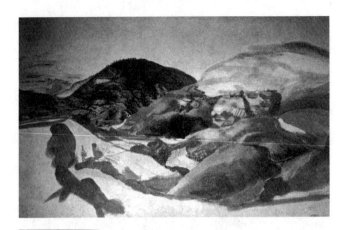

FIGURE 16.2 *Wehlsch Pirg* (Italian Mountain) by Albrecht Durer (approx. 1495).

Physical versus Emotional (Allie's Poem)

I could've listened to him for hours.
He was in his late 60s.
He'd had diabetes for the better part of his life
He was in the final stage of renal failure and for years and
years he had gone for dialysis three days a week for 4 or 5 hours a day.
When I first got to know him
I thought, "A man with diabetes and kidney failure."
I didn't think about anything else.
I considered him another "case"
but
there was way more.
He was a very intelligent guy and
He knew everything there was to know about
  Geography
When we talked,
He went into detail about how mountains form
and how there is the plateau
and how weather works with it
and then he went on to talk about how he had actually run like a radio show when he was
younger.
I was reminded to take the time to get to know my patients.
Holistic care
Getting to know the patient as a whole
because
We forget that the patients we have aren't just a physical body that needs to be taken care of.
They're an emotional body that needs to be taken care of, too.

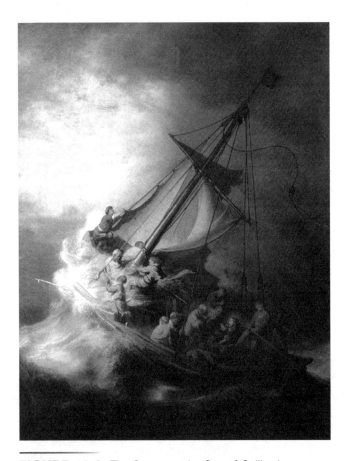

FIGURE 16.3 *The Storm on the Sea of Galilee* by Rembrandt (1633).

It's more physical sometimes and
We forget that we are "care providers."
We're there to care for them as a whole –
They have lived these wonderful lives and stuff.
It's the physical versus the emotional.

Emotions

Sisters (Boniva's Poem)

Severe dementia
She couldn't remember and
I kind of didn't expect her to
She was 94.

Who are you?
Who are you?
Who are you?
Every time she asks it,
It's stabbing her sister in the heart.
She knows that she knew all these things last week.
She can see her health deteriorating so quickly.

Her sister.
Her sister expressed
She was scared
She felt like everything was coming to an end because her sister –
     she's the oldest and
     she's the first one to die and
     she's the first one to get sick.

   "What's your favorite Bible verse?" she asked.
   "The Storm on the Sea of Galilee," I replied.

Jesus is in the boat with his disciples and the storm is raging around them and they all run in the back of the boat and plead, "Save us, save us. Please save us." Jesus wakes up and calms the storm and says, "If I'm in the back of the boat with you, why are you so scared?"

I told her about the story and I said, "Just remember that no matter how bad your health is deteriorating and what kind of storm is raging around you that there's always a purpose and you can see it when you're here and that Jesus is always in the back of your boat."

Fostering Change (Leigh's Poem)

She was 26.
She was an I.V. drug user.
She had an 18-month-old son.
She was playing with fire.
She hadn't been making changes
and was so close with death.
Her heart valve was damaged
And
She was going to have to undergo open-heart surgery.
I tried not to be so judgmental.
But
It was frustrating.
It was her first time in the hospital
So
I tried to be very compassionate and empathetic for her situation.
It's a new experience for her to know how to change.
I would've liked more connection with her.

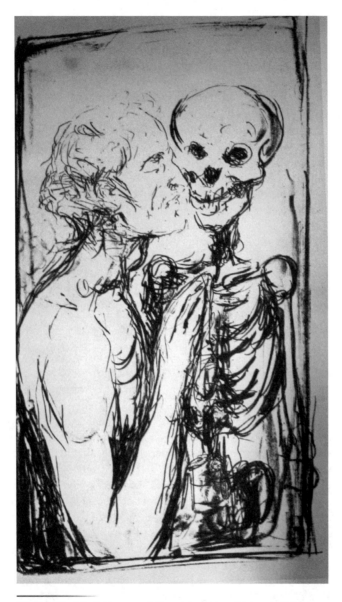

FIGURE 16.4 *Dance of Death* by Edvard Munch (1894).

Maybe she needed more motivation or support.
Maybe I could've been a causative agent in her change.
Hopefully, she will make a change.
Maybe she's learned now.
What she's doing is literally dancing with death.

DISCUSSION

The impact of arts-based instruction on clinical nursing students' perception of their own nursing practice is that integrating art into the clinical experience served as a useful curriculum tool to foster deep reflection. This change is demonstrated by the students' reflections that not only spanned the care they provided but looked closely at patient relationships through analysis of their own clinical practice. The use of Rose's (2001) visual critical methodology provided a framework from which to begin our interpretation of the words within our students' stories. We note, as Rose does, "interpreting images is just that, interpretation, not the discovery of their truth" (2001, p. 2). Therefore, rather than making validity claims in our discussion, we used relational criteria and face validity (Lather, 1986), sometimes referred to as member-checking, to demonstrate that the use of art in the clinical postconference setting can be beneficial.

Holistic care and the students' emotions related to their clinical practice were the most prominent themes within and across their stories. As evident in our re-presentation of data, emotions are woven throughout each of the poems. Because we are all emotional beings, it is often difficult for clinical nurses to separate their emotions from their practice (Scott, 2001). In this discussion, we look more closely at the individual themes of (1) holistic care provided by the students and (2) the emotions they experienced.

Holistic Care

Holistic care, which is one of the basic tenets of nursing practice, was discussed in the context of communication with patients and prioritization of care. Looking closely at Allie's poem, *Physical versus Emotional,* she first acknowledged that the care she had been providing was mostly physical in nature. She stated, "Patients aren't just a physical body that needs to be taken care of," indicating that her prioritization of care had changed. This change was apparent through her statement that her patients were "...an emotional body that needs to be taken care of, too." Prioritization of care is often thought about in terms of which physical ailment takes precedence when caring for a patient's condition. For the purpose of this study, prioritization of care is the students' realization that to care for the patient as a whole, it isn't unusual for a patient's mental or spiritual health to impact overall health just as much as physical health. Therefore, all of these dimensions should be considered when planning care for a patient.

The importance of effective communication is another well-studied area of nursing. Caris-Verhallen, Kerkstra, and Bensing (1997) recognize the central role of communication in nursing practice. One of the themes evident in the students' poems was communication. For example, in Boniva's poem, *Sisters,* the 94-year-old patient had severe dementia and could not remember her; she kept asking, "Who are you? Who are you? Who are you?" However, Boniva had an understanding about her patient and her condition and did not expect her to remember who she was. Another example is Louise's poem, *I Am Sure He Has a Story;* she realized that "I should've tried to talk to him more. I should have put more of an effort into just talking to him more, not necessarily trying to get something out of him." She reflected on the communication she didn't have the opportunity to have with her patient; hopefully, this will impact the care she gives in the future.

Emotions

According to Oakley (1992)

> ... the psychic dimension of emotional affectivity is the mental "tone" which affects us when we have an emotion, and which characteristically permeates our perceptions, desires and actions in ways which we are not always aware...in fact it is partly because of this perception-guiding function of emotional affectivity that emotions of various kinds can be seen as morally significant. (pp. 11–14)

Scott (2001) posits that "good nursing" implies the use of emotion in clinical practice. Smith (1991) studied the learning environment for student nurses and its relationship to quality of nursing care; she found the emotional aspects of caring associated with the nursing process to be an integral component of the student-patient relationship. The emotions that were evident through the students' reflections included loneliness, isolation, vulnerability, faith, hope, empathy, frustration, and regret. Christy's poem, not re-presented here, evokes feelings such as loneliness, isolation, and vulnerability. Christy showed empathy for her patient by pointing out that women must care for children and spouse, and have many other responsibilities. Faith was another emotion depicted in Boniva's poem, *Sisters*. It is important for nursing students to be able to recognize their emotions as well as the emotions of their patients to perceive the context and perspective of the situation more accurately (Scott, 2001). This activity enabled the students to verbalize not only their emotions but also the perceived emotions of their patients.

IMPLICATIONS FOR CLINICAL NURSING INSTRUCTION

We attempted to demonstrate that by using art as a medium for reflection, nursing students were able to express a variety of perspectives and meanings derived from their clinical experiences. The process of students engaging one another through the use of art fostered critical thinking as well as reflection in all the students involved. The use of art increased the students' ability to think more deeply about a patient they cared for or a situation that arose during the time they were caring for a patient. Through reflection on the semester, and with the students' descriptions of their experiences, this qualitative study allowed the clinical experience to become more meaningful. In their own words, students were able to compare works of art to the patients they cared for, which enabled them to reflectively process their views of their patients and themselves as caregivers. The impact of arts-based instruction on nursing students' perceptions of their own nursing practice allowed three themes to arise from their words: (1) holistic care, with subthemes communication and prioritization of care; (2) reflection, with subthemes self, patient, care; and (3) emotion, with subthemes faith, hope, empathy, frustration, and regret. All these themes are important for nursing students to understand and recognize when providing holistic care.

The use of art in the clinical postconference setting can be beneficial. There are key factors that should be present for this method to be effective. First, the students must be involved in the group and feel comfortable talking about feelings or situations they experienced throughout the semester. Second, there should be a variety of resources available to ensure that the student is able to make a connection between the artwork and an experience or patient encountered throughout the semester. Finally, the students must be acclimated to a teaching/learning environment that is more abstract and not quite as structured as the traditional classroom. According to Eisner (2002):

> Work in the arts also invites the development of a disposition to tolerate ambiguity, to explore what is uncertain, to exercise judgment free from prescriptive rules and procedures.... Work in the arts enables us to stop looking over our shoulders and to direct our attention inward to what we believe or feel. Such a disposition is at the root of individual autonomy. (p. 10)

Because of the nature of this clinical setting, the eight clinical nursing students had been working closely together for a period of six weeks. This particular clinical course incorporates a postconference meeting attended after each clinical day for a period of reflection. The students involved in this study were comfortable in the presence of each other, as well as their instructor, and very willing to take part in this nontraditional learning activity. This study should be considered by any nurse educator who is working to foster critical thinking, as well as the essential elements of holistic care.

References

Art. (2010). In *Oxford Dictionary Online.* Retrieved from http://www.oed.com/

Barone, T., & Eisner, E. (2006). Arts-based educational research. In J. L. Green, G. Camilli, & P. B. Elmore (Eds.), *Handbook of complementary methods in education research.* Washington, DC: American Educational Research Association.

Bevis, E. (1988). New directions for a new age. In National League for Nursing (Ed.), *Curriculum revolution: Mandate for change* (pp. 27–52). New York, NY: National League for Nursing.

Caris-Verhallen, W. M. C. M., Kerkstra, A., & Bensing, J. M. (1997). The role of communications in nursing care for elderly people: a review of the literature. *Journal of Advanced Nursing, 25*(5), 915–933.

Carper, B. (1978). Fundamental patterns of knowing in nursing. *Advances in Nursing Science, 1*(1), 13–23.

Casey, B. (2009). Arts-based inquiry in nursing education. *Contemporary Nurse: A Journal for the Australian Nursing Profession, 32*(1–2), 69–82.

Coffey, A., & Atkinson, P. (1996). *Making sense of qualitative data: Complementary research strategies.* Thousand Oaks, CA: Sage Publications.

Denzin, N. K., & Lincoln, Y. S. (Eds.). (1994). *The handbook of qualitative research.* Thousand Oaks, CA: Sage Publications.

Eisner, E. (2002). *The arts and the creation of mind.* New Haven, London: Yale University Press.

Glesne, C. (2007). *Becoming qualitative researchers: An introduction* (3rd ed.). White Plains, NY: Longman.

Grbich, C. (2007). *Qualitative data analysis: An introduction.* Thousand Oaks, CA: Sage Publications.

Hall, S. (1997). *Representations: Cultural representations and signifying practices.* London: Sage Publications.

Hammersly, M., & Atkinson, P. (1994). Ethnography and participant observation. In N. K. Denzin & Y. S. Lincoln (Eds.), *Handbook of qualitative research* (pp. 248–261). Thousand Oaks, CA: Sage Publications.

Hatch, J. A. (2002). *Doing qualitative research in education settings.* Albany, NY: State University of New York Press.

Inskeep, S. J., & Lisko, S. A. (2001). Teaching strategies: Alternative clinical nursing experience in an art gallery. *Nurse Educator, 26,* 117–119.

Jensen, A. & Curtis, M. (2008). A descriptive qualitative study of student learning in a psychosocial nursing class infused with art, literature, music, and film. *International Journal of Nursing Education Scholarship, 5*(1), Article 4.

Lather, P. (1986). Issues of validity in openly ideological research: Between a rock and a soft place. In Y. S. Lincoln & N. K. Denzin (Eds.), *Turning points in qualitative research: Tying knots in a handkerchief* (pp. 185–215). New York, NY: AltaMira Press.

Miles, M. B. & Huberman, A. M. (1994). *An expanded sourcebook: Qualitative data analysis* (2nd ed.). Thousand Oaks, CA: Sage Publications.

Noblit, G. W., Flores, S. Y., & Murillo, E. G. (Eds.). (2004). *Postcritical ethnography: Reinscribing critique.* Kresskill, NJ: Hampton Press, Inc.

Oakley, J. (1992). *Morality and the Emotions.* London, UK: Routledge.

Pellico, L. H., Friedlaender, L., & Fennie, K. P. (2009). Looking is not seeing: Using art to improve observational skills. *Journal of Nursing Education, 48*(11), 648–653.

Pillow, W. S. (2003). Confession, catharsis, or cure? Rethinking the uses of reflexivity as methodological power in qualitative research. *Qualitative Studies in Education, 16*(2), 175–196.

Ponto, J. A., Frost, M. H., & Thompson, R. (2003). Stories of breast cancer through art. *Oncology Nursing Forum Online, 30*(6), 1007–1013.

Rose, G. (2001). *Visual methodologies: An introduction to the interpretation of visual materials.* London: Sage Publications.

Scott, P. A. (2001). Emotion, moral perception, and nursing practice. *Nursing Philosophy, 1*(2), 123–133.

Smith, R. L., Bailey, M., Hydo, S. K., Lepp, M., Mews, S., & Timm, S. (2004). All the voices in the room: Integrating humanities in nursing education. *Nursing Education Perspectives, 25*, 278–283.

Smith, P. (1991). The nursing process: Raising the profile of emotional care in nurse training. *Journal of Advanced Nursing, 16*, 74–81.

Staricoff, R. (2006). Arts in health: The value of evaluation. *Journal of the Royal Society for the Promotion of Health, 126*(3), 116–120.

Strauss, A. L. (1987). *Qualitative analysis for social scientists.* Cambridge: Cambridge University Press.

Valiga, T. M., & Bruderle, E. R. (1997). *Using the arts and humanities to teach nursing: A creative approach.* New York, NY: Springer.

Weick, K. E. (1976). Educational organizations as loosely coupled systems. *Administrative Science Quarterly, 21*(1), 1–18.

Whitman, B. L., & Rose, J. (2003). Using art to express a personal philosophy of nursing. *Nurse Educator, 28*(4), 166–169.

17

Teaching Thinking in Nursing Using Art

Priscilla K. Gazarian, PhD, RN

In today's world, our senses are bombarded with information from numerous sources simultaneously, making *applying* and *evaluating* information more important than *having* information. Nurses work in environments in which they are presented with multiple bits and pieces of information. They are obliged to make sense of it in pursuit of the goal of providing safe and reliable care. Learning to think and evaluate information in real time becomes a necessary skill for nurses. To meet this challenge, professional nurses must develop expert clinical reasoning skills (Burritt & Steckel, 2009). Educational approaches that foster thinking skills and creativity are necessary (Benner, Sutphen, Leonard, & Day, 2010). The use of art interpretation as a teaching strategy is one approach that fosters the development of thinking in new ways as well as an appreciation for multiple perspectives (Ewing & Hayden-Miles, 2011).

Traditionally, nurse educators have focused on teaching methods such as critical thinking exercises or case studies to develop and make explicit clinical reasoning. Viewing and interpreting works of art can be a useful activity in developing awareness of reasoning skills. The learning activity described in this chapter seeks to develop students' awareness of their thinking by using works of art as an information source. Students were asked to extract meaning from pieces of art using various prompts. The activity required students to examine their thinking related to the work of art. Classroom discussion aided in revealing the presence of preconceptions and individual perceptions and their effect on reasoning in various ways.

THEORETICAL BACKGROUND

The use of the arts and humanities in nursing education is well documented and supported by the *Essentials of Baccalaureate Education for Professional Nursing Practice* (American Association of Colleges of Nursing [AACN], 2008). Carper's (1978) seminal paper on patterns of knowing in nursing created the groundwork for nurse educators to give equal prominence to aesthetic knowledge in curricula traditionally dominated by empiric knowledge.

Nurse educators have used the arts and humanities within a nursing curriculum in various ways. Several authors have reported the use of entire courses devoted to art interpretation and creation (Blomqvist, Pitkala, & Routasalo, 2007; Casey, 2009; Darbyshire, 1994). These courses addressed a range of learning goals such as fostering personal creativity; developing critical, reflective, interpretive, and analytical thinking; developing empathy; and understanding the experience of loneliness, suffering, chronic pain, miscarriage, and disability. Nurse educators also use the arts and humanities for specific assignments within a course. For example, Pellico and colleagues described the use of a museum visit to develop observational skills as part of a physical assessment course (Pellico, Friedlaender, & Fennie, 2009), while Inskeep and Lisko (2001) reported on the use of a museum visit to teach the use of nursing diagnosis.

The specific assignment described in this chapter sought to develop awareness of reasoning strategies among nursing students within a capstone clinical decision-making course through the interpretation of art. The assignment is a synthesis of ideas from Visual Thinking Strategies (VTS) (Visual Thinking Strategies, 2010) and Tanner's clinical judgment model (Tanner, 2006). VTS is a curriculum based on over 30 years of research by Abigail Housen (Longhenry, 2005). VTS uses art to develop skills in thinking, communication, observation, and visual literacy. It is a learner-centered approach that uses facilitated discussions to expose diverse thinking and problem-solving abilities (Yenawine, 1998). The curriculum is widely used in pre-kindergarten through high school settings, medical education, preservice teacher training, and corporate and public sector staff development (Visual Thinking Strategies, 2010). Although the use of VTS with nursing students has not previously been reported, VTS principles, which center on developing creative, critical, and independent thinking, are congruent with the goals of this particular course and assignment.

Housen reported on the Byron Study "Methods for Museum Education," a 5-year longitudinal study that sought to investigate the effects of VTS on aesthetic growth and transfer of VTS-learned skills (Housen, 2001). The findings from the study presented here support the assumption that critical thinking skills developed through VTS do transfer to nonart objects and subjects (Housen, 2001). Building on the premise that the thinking skills developed through VTS are transferable, the assignment described here uses works of art to expose the students' thinking strategies, and then have them apply this new awareness of thinking strategies to thinking like a nurse.

Thinking like a nurse, as described by Tanner in her model of clinical judgment (2006), is comprised of three methods of reasoning. These include analytical processes, intuition, and narrative thinking.

- Analytic processes are systematic and rational, involving breaking a situation down into parts or elements and weighing alternatives against one other.

- Intuitive reasoning is described as pattern recognition developed through experience, allowing an immediate understanding of a situation.

- Narrative thinking allows humans to infer causation, make sense, or explain what they see in terms of the human experience.

Nurses use these types of reasoning to varying degrees according to the context of clinical situations (Tanner, 2006). This assignment allowed nursing students to bring awareness and attention to their reasoning related to a nonnursing subject, the interpretation of a piece of art. The use of a nonnursing subject, such as art interpretation, was instrumental in the success of this assignment. Students felt open to share ideas about their reasoning related to art, rather than feeling a responsibility to know the answer related to a nursing topic.

PROJECT DESCRIPTION

The purpose of this assignment was to use a common and accessible experience—viewing pieces of art—to expose students' reasoning processes and increase their awareness of those processes. The learning objectives were to apply observation and different types of reasoning to describe and interpret a work of art.

As part of the assignment design, works of art appropriate for the assignment were chosen. The Museum of Fine Arts, Boston, offers a Community Education Department with staff willing to assist in the selection of appropriate pieces. In collaboration with the museum's manager of school and teacher partnerships, pieces were selected based on a few broad criteria. First, each picture needed to include a human subject given that narrative reasoning focuses on the human experience. Second, abstract art was avoided, as interpretation of this type of art tends to be difficult for students with limited art education. Last, pieces were selected from the modern era, when artists began to depict scenes of everyday life to which the students could relate. Expert consultation was helpful in selecting pieces with broad appeal. A list of the selected paintings was provided to the students that included the title of each work, its catalog number, and its gallery location. Students viewed the paintings as an out-of-class assignment.

Prior to visiting the museum, the students were asked to read Tanner's *Thinking Like a Nurse* (2006) in preparation for applying the three types of reasoning she described: intuitive, analytic, and narrative. In completing the assignment, students were to carefully observe each of the six pieces. Students were instructed to closely examine the paintings, to examine them from a distance, then to look at them from different distances and angles to encourage active observation. Students were asked to note their thoughts in response to the following prompts:

- **Intuitive Reasoning:** Describe your immediate impression of this picture. What interests you about this picture? What feelings does it evoke?

- **Analytic Reasoning:** What do you see specifically that leads you to these impressions? Describe your observations using evidence to back up observations.

- **Narrative Reasoning:** Tell the story about what's going on in this picture.

Students selected the one painting that most interested them individually from the group of six and, prior to class, wrote a one- to two-paragraph response to each of the three types of reasoning.

Class discussion of the exercise was facilitated by preparing a PowerPoint® presentation with images of the paintings provided by the museum. Because students had the opportunity to ponder the paintings and commit their responses to paper prior to class, each had some remarks to contribute to the in-class discussion. Each painting was discussed in turn and the students offered their ideas on each of the three types of reasoning.

The students shared their reflections in class discussion and revealed a great diversity in their preconceptions and perceptions, as well as how they used various types of reasoning to respond to the paintings. The following is an example of the similarities and differences in the three types of reasoning shared by the students related to one of the paintings.

Thirteen students chose to write about Renoir's "The Dance at Bougival," a large impressionistic painting of a couple dancing at an outdoor café. In response to the first question, students overwhelmingly responded to the size of the canvas, the bright colors, and the lively brushstrokes. However, the group was evenly split in their initial response, with some feeling that this was a romantic and joyful dance between a young couple in love and others feeling there was unease between the two dance partners. As they answered the prompt about analytical reasoning, the students produced evidence to support their individual initial impressions. Evidence they offered included observations such as the facial expression of the woman, the woman was not looking at the man, the man was not dressed as elegantly as the woman or the other men in the painting's background, and a ring on the woman's left hand. Although several students noted the woman's facial expression, those whose impression was that this was a young couple in love analyzed her expression as shy with a hint of pleasure. Those whose impression was of unease analyzed her expression as uncomfortable, with averted eyes, turning away from her partner. Last, the students tried to make sense of the painting in terms of human experience such as: "Her averted face is because this is a forbidden love and they are from different social classes." To some, the couple is married; to others, the woman who wears a ring is married, but to someone else. Some saw the woman as simply fulfilling the role expected of her as the shy and desired woman.

Despite their diverse opinions, the students were all viewing the very same painting. The in-class discussion made evident that each person's response to each piece of art was unique and the challenge was to remain open to new interpretations of situations.

Students were able to relate these ideas to clinical situations. For instance, students shared ideas about differing interpretations of patient body language and the implications of those interpretations for patient care. A patient's inability to make eye contact may be interpreted as respect, fear, avoidance, or dishonesty. The students' challenge was to become aware of their preconceptions and interpretations and be open to a new interpretation as further assessment data were collected.

Another popular painting was Sargent's "Mrs. Fiske Warren and Daughter, Rachel." One student related that she was drawn to this painting because of the recent loss of her mother and had been reflecting on the mother–daughter relationship. She felt that the painting evoked comforting feelings of closeness and adoration between a mother and her child. In contrast, other students had a completely different impression of this painting. One saw the mother as uncomfortable, fidgeting, and the daughter offering her mother support. Yet another student saw the mother as stoic, rigid, unloving, and not caring. Class discussion related to these various perceptions illustrated Tanner's point that judgment is influenced by what the nurse brings to the situation in terms of past experiences (Tanner, 2006).

As students shared their interpretations of the paintings, it was not difficult to transition to thinking in clinical situations. As a group, the students were able to bring awareness to patterns in their thinking individually and collectively such as how preconceptions and perception affect reasoning, how one can make assumptions in thinking, how some notice certain details about a patient assessment while others notice something different, and how who we are as individuals affects what we perceive.

EVALUATION

The submitted written responses, class discussion, and anonymous student feedback were used to evaluate the exercise as a learning experience. The written responses required students to address the three types of reasoning. The goal was not whether they presented a right or wrong answer but to present their thinking about the art in three different ways. All of the students (100%) were able to address all three types of reasoning in their writing. The class discussion was rich and informative, exposing a great diversity of thinking, with students verbalizing a new awareness of reasoning in clinical situations. End-of-class and course evaluations included comments specific to this assignment such as:

- "This was a good way to extrapolate information from a still piece in much the same way as we do when initially viewing a patient."
- "An engaging way to get us to think about how we think."
- "This assignment helps us to better understand how we make our decisions and why we reach our conclusions."
- "It was interesting to review all our interpretations in class as a base for discussion regarding patient scenarios."

Students unanimously recommended future use of this assignment. Students viewed the experience as fun and a great opportunity to explore the art museum with the goal to think about their thinking. Related to learning to think, students commented that the assignment:

- "Broadened my perspectives."
- "Made me think about the ways that I make clinical judgments and the assumption and biases that come into practice."
- Was "a good exercise to look at your thinking processes."

CONCLUSIONS

After viewing, responding to, and discussing works of art, students gained new awareness of reasoning strategies and postulated how that awareness could be transferred to thinking and problem solving in caring for patients. The uniqueness of this assignment lies in first bringing attention to thinking about a nonnursing subject. Looking at art allows each person the freedom to articulate what they see, not what they think should be the right answer. Asking students to commit to writing their thoughts about a piece of art from three different perspectives brings attention to their cognitive processing, which is often unnoticed in everyday life.

When sharing their reflection on the paintings as a group, students witnessed powerful evidence of how preconceptions, perceptions, and individual circumstances affect the way one thinks. This exercise is a powerful way to encourage student nurses to be open-minded, observant, inquisitive, and careful thinkers. The nursing profession is challenged to transform the way new nurses are educated as increasing emphasis is placed on clinical judgment skills (Benner et al., 2010). Innovative and evidenced-based teaching methods aimed at developing and refining clinical reasoning skills are necessary. Future researchers might study how VTS methods are best used in nursing and their effect on learning and practice outcomes.

References

American Association of Colleges of Nursing (AACN). (2008). *The Essentials of Baccalaureate Education for Professional Nursing Practice.* Washington DC: Author.

Benner, P., Sutphen, M., Leonard, V., & Day, L. (2010). *Educating nurses: A call for radical transformation.* Stanford, CA: Jossey-Bass.

Blomqvist, L., Pitkala, K., & Routasalo, P. (2007). Images of loneliness: Using art as an educational method in professional training. *Journal of Continuing Education in Nursing, 38*(2), 89–93.

Burritt, J., & Steckel, C. (2009). Supporting the learning curve for contemporary nursing practice. *Journal of Nursing Administration, 39*(11), 479–484.

Carper, B. (1978). Fundamental patterns of knowing in nursing. *Advances in Nursing Science, 1*(1), 13–24.

Casey, B. (2009). Arts-based inquiry in nursing education. *Contemporary Nurse: A Journal for the Australian Nursing Profession, 32*(1–2), 69–82.

Darbyshire, P. (1994). Understanding caring through arts and humanities: A medical/nursing humanities approach to promoting alternative experiences of thinking and learning. *Journal of Advanced Nursing, 19*(5), 856–863.

Ewing, B., & Hayden-Miles, M. (2011). Narrative pedagogy and art interpretation. *Journal of Nursing Education, 50*(4), 211.

Housen, A. (2001, April 10–14, 2001). *Methods for assessing transfer from an art-viewing program.* Paper presented at the Annual Meeting of the American Educational Research Association, Seattle, WA.

Inskeep, S. J., & Lisko, S. A. (2001). Teaching strategies: Alternative clinical nursing experience in an art gallery. *Nurse Educator, 26*(3), 117–119.

Longhenry, S. (2005). Thinking through art at the Boston Museum of Fine Arts. *School Arts: The Art Education Magazine for Teachers, 104*(7), 56.

Pellico, L. H., Friedlaender, L., & Fennie, K. P. (2009). Looking is not seeing: Using art to improve observational skills. *Journal of Nursing Education, 48*(11), 648–653.

Tanner, C. A. (2006). Thinking like a nurse: A research-based model of clinical judgment in nursing. *Journal of Nursing Education, 45*(6), 204–211.

Visual Thinking Strategies. (2010). Retrieved from www.vtshome.org

Yenawine, P. (1998). Visual art and student-centered discussions. *Theory into Practice, 37*(4), 314–321.

18

Blogging:
A Tool for Reflective Learning
in Nursing Education

Phyllis Ann Solari-Twadell, PhD, RN, FAAN
Monique Ridosh, MSN, RN
Sarah Brittain Dysart, MA
Gail Hanson, MSN, RN

The nursing literature notes the use of a blog (short for "web log," online online environments that provide space and organization for journal-style electronic entries) for faculty development, continuing nursing education, and nursing informatics education (Shaffer, Lackey, & Bolling, 2006; Billings, 2009; Brixey & Warren, 2009). Blogging creates a learning opportunity for debate and reflection of ideas (Burke & Oomen-Earley, 2008). The benefit of using a blog for health education includes "providing more information for engagement and conversation with this added user engagement promoting messages and ideas that are processed and more fully internalized instead of merely communicated" (Hanson, Thackeray, Barnes, Neiger, & McIntyre, 2008, p. 160).

The study reported in this chapter involved three sections of one freshman course delivered in a seminar format that met eight times throughout the semester; it provided the context for the experiential learning cycle. The objective of the student writing assignment—both through blogging and on paper—was to develop insight and invite the student to engage in critical thinking.

A requirement of the course is eight hours of service-learning experience in a designated location. The service locations included a homeless shelter for men, women, and children; a children's hospital; and a skilled nursing facility. Students were assigned six reflection questions that related to the service being provided (see Box 18.1 for sample reflection questions). Faculty developed their own reflections related to each of the six questions in a blog that was open to students for reading and comments. Once students participated in the blog, they developed their own one- to two-page reflection papers related to each of the six questions. These papers were then collected as part of the face-to-face seminar.

THEORETICAL UNDERPINNINGS

Kolb and Kolb (2009) highlight the interdisciplinary widespread application of experiential learning theory spanning 40 years. The philosophical underpinning of radical

BOX 18.1 SAMPLE REFLECTION QUESTIONS ON THE SERVICE-LEARNING EXPERIENCE

- **Serving the Poor:** The Jesuits identify service as one of the primary characteristics of their tradition. How does serving the poor fit within the Jesuit tradition? What are some of your feelings, concerns, or anticipation in serving the poor? How does providing service for this population fit with your vocation of nursing within the Jesuit tradition?
- **Being Unattended:** Sociologists noted at one time that Skid Row men in the United States had been carefully and extensively studied for more than 80 years and information regarding them as a population is readily available. Homeless women, however, seem to be more of a mystery. What are some of the implications of this statement? What feelings do you experience in reflecting on this information? What are some of the differences for a man versus a woman being homeless and unattended?
- **Being Isolated:** The elderly are at risk of isolation related to changes in environment and support systems. As you interact with the population, you will have an opportunity to understand how the environment and frequency of contact with support systems impact residents' feelings of loneliness or isolation. What impact has your presence made while serving? What other feelings and thoughts come to mind for you in serving this population?
- **Being Mentally Ill:** All people have their own story, which has contributed to where they work, what they are passionate about, where they are living, and the service they offer to others. Each individual who is homeless and mentally ill has his or her own story as well. What are some of the factors that could contribute to the mentally ill being homeless? As future health care professionals, how can you reach out to this population and make a difference?
- **Being Invisible:** The elderly population is vulnerable to neglect. What does it mean to you to be present but to be invisible to others? Have you ever felt invisible? If not, what do you think it might feel like to be present and yet seem to be invisible to others? What kind of feelings can result? What might be some of the outcomes if you are not "seen" by others or seen as a threat rather than a person?
- **Being Under-resourced:** The elderly are often unable to negotiate the bewildering bureaucratic health care maze. Others know it so well that they abuse the health care services offered. What are some of the obstacles that you think the elderly may encounter in trying to access health care services? Can you imagine what being poor and sick would be like for yourself? How would you feel if you had no means to access health care?
- **Caring and Service:** Questions to ask yourself are: What service have I provided as part of this course? What meaning did it have for me? What ethical issues were raised through this service opportunity? What meaning did this service have for the recipient? How did this experience broaden my understanding of myself? How did this experience relate to my understanding of nursing, caring, and service?

empiricism grounds experiential learning theory and learning cycle development. These theorists use a meta-cognitive model to describe how the concepts of the theory of experiential learning can guide development of learning capacity (Kolb & Kolb, 2009). They further characterize the learning cycle as experiencing, reflecting, thinking, and acting. The monitoring and control of the learning process model at the object level leads to effective learning at the meta level. Concepts of the experiential learning theory include a learning self-identity, the spiral learning process, learning style, learning space, and learning flexibility. Requesting students to read faculty blogs, reflect on those writings, think about their own response, and then compose their reflection is application of this learning cycle.

Lisko and O'Dell (2010) describe the application of Kolb's theory of experiential learning with technology as a strategy to promote critical thinking. Learning occurs as a continuous process whereby "knowledge is created by transforming experience into existing cognitive frameworks, thus changing the way a person thinks and behaves" (Lisko & O'Dell, 2010, p. 106). Practice integration occurs when experiences are grasped through "apprehension" (practice) or "comprehension" (abstract conceptualization). The learning that occurs as experience is transformed through the process of "extension" (active participation) or "intention" (reflection). The learning process encompasses each step of the cycle: (a) concrete experience, (b) reflection, (c) abstract conceptualization, and (d) active experimentation (Lisko & O'Dell, 2010).

Scheffer and Rubenfeld (2000) define critical thinking as "habits of the mind" and "skills" in nursing with affective and cognitive components. In a five-round Delphi study, an international panel of nurse educators, nurse researchers, and nurse clinicians discerned critical thinking habits of the mind to include confidence, contextual perspective, creativity, flexibility, inquisitiveness, intellectual integrity, intuition, open-mindedness, perseverance, and reflection. Skills include analyzing, discriminating, logical reasoning, applying standards, information seeking, predicting, and transforming knowledge (Scheffer & Rubenfeld, 2000). The assigning of six reflections using the same process was intentional in creating "habits of the mind" for the students to enhance critical thinking.

METHODS

The researchers designed a descriptive qualitative study to explore the use of a blog in a freshman nursing course to which they were assigned as faculty. The faculty sought and received approval from the institutional review board (IRB) of the sponsoring university. A consent form was required for students to participate in the study. Use of the blog was encouraged by faculty, but not mandatory for the students. Two different rubrics were developed to facilitate the evaluation of both the reflection papers and the students' blog entries. The rubrics were used to evaluate the students' ability to reflect. Criteria used for paper assessment were: (a) inclusion of concepts noted in reflection questions; (b) grammar, punctuation, spelling; (c) examples from own life experience; and (d) identified insight or new learning about self through reflection. Criteria used for blog entry assessment were: (a) comprehension of blog content; (b) clarity and organization of entry; and (c) writing, grammar, spelling. The intent of the rubrics was to begin to evaluate the habits of the mind and skills of critical thinking (see Tables 18.1 and 18.2).

Reflection papers and the related blog comments that pertained to the reflection questions were used to evaluate the effectiveness of the blog in impacting the quality of

TABLE 18.1

Reflective Papers Rubric

Ranking/Criteria	Exemplary	Good	Satisfactory	Poor
Inclusion of concepts noted in reflection questions	Responds to concepts raised that question self-understanding	Responds to questions noted in reflection questions; however, there is limited evidence of self-understanding.	Responds to reflection questions.	Attempts to respond to reflection questions but misses the intent of the reflection questions.
Grammar, punctuation, spelling	No grammar, punctuation, or spelling errors	One grammar, punctuation, or spelling error.	Two grammar, punctuation, or spelling errors.	Three grammar, punctuation, or spelling errors.
Inclusion of good examples from own life experience	Includes pertinent examples from own life related to reflection topic and questions.	Responds to reflection questions and refers to life experience but does not link experiences directly to the reflection topic.	Responds to reflection questions.	Does not respond to reflection questions.
Identification of insight or new learning about self through reflection	Identifies an understanding of self from a new perspective.	Responds to reflection questions; however, this response does not result in any new understanding of self.	Responds to reflection questions.	Does not respond to reflection questions.

the reflection paper. The evaluation of the reflection papers and blog entries was completed following the assignment of final grades. Student evaluation forms provided comments and feedback. These evaluation forms were completed at the end of the semester. Box 18.2 provides a sample evaluation form.

The freshman students in a nursing-as-service class received documents outlining the purpose of the blog, directions, and a link to the blog site. Students were informed that commentary posted to the blog was publicly available to those who knew the address. The use of the blog was introduced and discussed in each seminar section. Students were encouraged to use the blog in the development of their reflection papers. The reflection

TABLE 18.2

Blog Entry Rubric

Dimension	Accomplished	Competent	Developing	Novice
Comprehension	Clearly understood faculty posting and responded clearly to ideas noted in faculty posting, providing examples from own life.	Expressed understanding of faculty posting. Responded to some ideas noted in faculty posting, but does not include examples from own life.	Commented on faculty posting but did not respond to ideas expressed by faculty or give examples from own life.	Entered a comment; however, the comment did not relate to the posting by faculty or provide examples from own life.
Clarity and organization	Ideas clearly written, well organized, and stated with clear examples.	Ideas are presented; however, they may not be clearly expressed.	Ideas are presented but are lacking in organization.	There are brief comments entered, but they are not organized.
Grammar, punctuation, spelling	No grammar, punctuation, or spelling errors.	Minor errors in grammar, punctuation, or spelling.	More than two errors in grammar, punctuation, or spelling.	Consistent errors in grammar, punctuation, or spelling.

paper assignments were due at specified times during the semester. Consent forms were distributed for student review and signature. It was emphasized that student participation in the study would not affect the grade received for the course.

Faculty posted their responses to the reflection questions on the blog one to two weeks before each reflection paper was due. The students were informed when faculty posted their submissions and invited to use the blog. Students were encouraged to read faculty posts and record their thoughts following review of the faculty reflection. Following the blogging activity, students submitted their reflection papers. The papers were graded within one to two weeks of submission. Faculty did not read responses to the blog before grading student reflection papers. At the end of the course, grades were submitted based on the work the students had completed in accordance with course assignments.

ANALYSIS

Four of the research team members analyzed the data. First, students who consented to participate were identified. The blog entries completed by students who consented to

BOX 18.2 SAMPLE EVALUATION TOOL FOR BLOG USE

Evaluation of the Use of the Blog

1. Did you use the blog in preparing your reflections for the "Nursing as Service" class?

   ____**Yes** Please proceed with the remainder of the evaluation.

   ____**No** Please explain why you did not use the blog to assist in preparation of your reflection papers on the lines following this question.

   _____
   _____
   _____
   _____
   _____

2. What did you find to be most helpful in using the blog as part of preparing your reflections for the Nursing as Service Course?

   _____
   _____
   _____
   _____
   _____

3. How do you think use of the blog could be improved to assist in preparation for the reflection papers assignments?

   _____
   _____
   _____
   _____
   _____

4. Additional Comments

   _____
   _____
   _____
   _____

participate in the study were analyzed by each member of the research team independently using the same rubric. Once this evaluation was completed, the team members discussed their scores and rationale. Dialog among researchers continued until consensus on the assigned score was reached. Next, the corresponding student reflection paper was reviewed independently by each researcher and a score for the paper assigned. Again, the team discussed the score and rationale of each reflection paper and came to consensus on the assigned score. The score for each student's blog entry was then compared with both the score given on the paper and the grade earned in the class. Students' blog evaluation forms were then reviewed. Comments from students who had signed consent forms were organized into common themes. Nonparticipating student comments were excluded from the study.

FINDINGS

Eleven students used the blog as part of this class; these students signed the consent form to participate and made entries on the blog. The total number of blog entries was 35. The scores using the blog rubric and the reflection rubric did not show significant changes in the quality of the reflection paper. In responding to one reflection question, Being Mentally Ill, five students had similar ranking of blog entry and reflection paper, mostly in the range of accomplished (blog entry) and exemplary (reflection). The following is an example of an accomplished student blog entry.

> Being from a really small town, I don't have much experience with homeless people. Moving to the city has opened my eyes to the fact that homeless people are not just dirty old people who want your money to buy drugs. I've come to realize that many mentally homeless people are that way because they do not have the capability to function as a "normal" person within society, as you said. I think we need to listen to their stories and get them off the streets.

Table 18.3 shows a sample of these results. A difference in quality is detected in one paper ranging from poor (reflection) to developing (blog entry). The following is an example of a developing blog entry.

> Upon reflecting on many of these women's situations, I guess I never thought about their ability to take the medication; whether stolen or lack of proper times. This reminds me of something my mom said one day after working at the community clinic, she said that they may have medication, but see no pressing need to take it as faithfully as needed. These situations lead me to think that the homeless also need health education for what and why they're taking the medications they are taking. I can see now that medication can't cure everything, rather health professionals need to start instructing and offering more services to help these people stay on top of their treatment which I guess opens a whole new can of worms for getting the treatment out to them.

TABLE 18.3

Data for Reflection—Being Mentally III

Student	Blog Comment Rubric Rating	Reflection Rubric Rating
1	Accomplished	Exemplary
2	Developing	Poor with good grammar
3	Accomplished	Exemplary
4	Accomplished	Good
5	Accomplished	Exemplary

In one example, the student handed in the reflection paper and then made an entry on the blog; the writing of the paper and associated reflections on the subject positively impacted the quality of the blog entry. The combined use of the blog and the reflection paper may have stimulated critical thinking for the beginning nursing student.

Themes from the student evaluations included learning to reflect and learning through modeling. Feedback from students suggested that students not only used blog entries written by faculty as a model for structuring their own reflection papers, but they extended their thinking on the topic. This illustrated that these beginning freshman students learned by examining the process shaped by an expert faculty. This was evident in the analysis of the papers; many students followed a structure and flow that was very similar to the posts completed by faculty on the blog. Students affirmed that being able to read an instructor's perspective gave them insight and a further understanding of the expected outcome for the assignment. One student stated, "Some of the reflections I knew exactly what I was going to write about." Other comments included: "I had no idea where to start" and "After reading some of the blogs, it gave me insight and in a way, guided me to answer the reflection questions correctly." The following are examples of student evaluation responses.

> Relaxing my mind and letting me focus on what I needed to reflect on including the questions given to us. I definitely opened up while writing, which made me more comfortable with writing down what goes through my mind and feelings. I think reflecting, knowing who you are, and comfortable with sharing yourself are major components of being a great nurse. Also, I wanted to read what other students and professors had to say on the matter presented to us.
>
> The reflections gave me the time, I wouldn't have otherwise spent on my experiences, to actually process what I had learned from the situations I was placed in. I never just wrote what I knew the teacher wanted to hear from me like I do in many other classes, because I had taken reflection time.
>
> It helped me relate my ideas to others and to understand that I wasn't the only one going through a transformation during the course. I could read and understand other people's opinions about the service that we were doing and understand the differences in past and present experiences of service.

DISCUSSION

The blog evaluation forms indicated an overall positive response to the study. The use of the developed rubrics and standardized approach to evaluation of writing did not yield significant difference in the quality of writing in the reflection papers.

Theory of Experiential Learning

The learning process is facilitated by creating space and flexibility to guide the student through the reflection process in the blog. Service learning and a prior knowledge of a topic form the concrete experience. In reflective observation, the student makes sense of the experience as perspectives are considered by participation in the seminar and review of the blog. Abstract conceptualization occurs as students think about ideas based on concrete experience and reflective observation. As students construct their written response in the reflection paper, the transformation of learning is completed. Students are guided through each step of Kolb's learning cycle to experience, reflect, think, and act.

Themes of Ways of Knowing

Learning to Reflect

Studies indicate that engaging students in activities that promote critical reflection can lead to deeper learning, including the improved ability to synthesize, analyze, and, over time, apply to situations they encounter (Strampel & Oliver, 2007). Other research considers reflection as "the creation of meaning and conceptualization from experience and the potentiality to look at things as other than they are" (Brockbank & McGill, 1998, p. 64). The ability to look beyond the stated word and create meaning is significant to this blogging study. Students stated that reading the entries on the blog and commenting helped them initiate the process of reflection. One student stated that the blog helped to, "put thoughts into perspective and expand in areas I thought were irrelevant to the topics given." Students commented that using the blog prompted them to process and internalize what they had learned from their experiences in the course. Another student remarked that the blog facilitated "reflecting, knowing who you are, and comfort with sharing yourself," which are skills required of any successful nurse.

Learning through Modeling

Students valued both model blog entries that instructors posted and the comments from their fellow students. Both types of assistance are characteristic of cognitive apprenticeship, an approach to learning that introduces students to new concepts via participation in authentic activity in their field of study. Cognitive apprenticeship refers to both the modeling of processes that experts use in their day-to-day practice as well as "the focus of the learning-through-guided-experience on cognitive and metacognitive, rather than physical, skills and processes" (Collins, Brown, & Newman, 1989, p. 457).

Strengths

The ethos and educational objectives of the university, including a published document developed by the university describing transformational education, provided a strong direction for employing learning strategies that reinforced use of reflection. The objectives and subject matter of the course also lent to the introduction and use of a blog. This assignment and the use of the blog provided affirmation for the students on what they were experiencing.

From the beginning of the academic year, the three faculty involved in teaching the course collaborated and maintained high-level communication with each other. The research team, which included the three nursing faculty members and one staff from the Office of Learning Technologies and Assessment, maintained consistent, clear communication. Open, honest, and clear communication was key. The fact that the university provided resources on the use of blogs and other Web 2.0 modalities made the study possible, as the nursing faculty themselves needed significant support in their initial use of the technology.

The student evaluation tool (Box 18.2), comprising open-ended questions, provided valuable feedback. Student comments on the use of the blog illustrated the value of the blog in providing faculty role modeling and stimulating critical thinking.

LIMITATIONS

The course had a seminar format with eight face-to-face meetings. Because seminar times varied among the three courses, consent forms were distributed and collected at different times. Two faculty members collected the consent forms on the same day they were distributed; one asked to have them returned during a subsequent class, which yielded fewer consent form submissions. Another setback involved the inaccessibility of the blog technology at the beginning of the course; this was relatively easy to remedy once the correct link to the blog was obtained and distributed.

Although the intention was to limit blog access to enrolled students and faculty, some individuals who were not part of the course accessed the blog. This presented some concern for investigators; could the intrusion of nonenrolled students inhibit honest reflective postings by participating students? An additional limitation of the study was the inability to access statistics on how many students entered the blog, read the posted material, but did not contribute any entries. One final condition that may have impacted the study was the distribution of the student evaluation tool. The evaluation was emailed several weeks after the conclusion of the course rather than distributed during the last face-to-face seminar. This delay may have limited the return rate of the evaluation form.

CONCLUSIONS

Although data received as a result of this descriptive qualitative study indicated little effect of the use of the blog on the quality of the reflection paper, this study proved valuable from several other perspectives. The study provided evidence that the use of a blog enhanced the learning experience for students in several distinct ways:

1. It helped students further understand the ethos and educational objectives of this university.
2. It provided faculty with feedback regarding how to make the reflective-writing experience more useful for students in future iterations of the course.
3. It indicated the value of the blog in fostering critical thinking.

Findings of this blogging study are supported by the work of Zeng and Harris (2005), who reported that 60 percent of the participants in a baccalaureate health information management course agreed that use of a blog can serve as a strategy for reflective thinking and writing. This study validates blogging in the context of a nursing education course as a theory-based learning strategy for reflecting-writing practice.

Habits of the Mind and Skills

The structure and process of this course facilitated student development of critical thinking by teaching habits of the mind and skills. Habits of the mind that this strategy promotes include thinking in context, flexibility to change ideas or adapt behaviors, inquisitiveness, intuition, open-mindedness that facilitates being receptive to other's perspectives, and being aware of one's own values. Skills that this activity promotes include analysis, application of standards, and logical reasoning. Collins et al. (1989) established that cognitive apprenticeship involves the externalization of processes that are often carried out internally. They assert that, "Observing the processes by which an expert listener or reader thinks and practicing these skills under the guidance of the expert can teach students to learn on their own more skillfully" (Collins et al., 1989, p. 459). Furthermore, they state that "cognitive apprenticeship teaching methods are designed to bring these tacit processes into the open, where students can observe, enact, and practice them with help from the teacher and from other students" (Collins et al., 1989, p. 458). Student comments in this study were consistent, noting that they found it helpful to read about the experiences of their instructors and peers and compare their personal experiences with those of others. One student stated, "I enjoyed reading the professors' reflections because I gained their knowledge and also gained a new respect for them and the nursing profession as a whole." Another student commented, "I could read and understand other people's opinions about the service that we were doing and understand the differences in past and present experiences of service."

Reinforcing the Ethos of the University

The emphasis on reflection inherent in the learning strategy in this course was intended to be a direct manifestation of the university's mission of "working to expand knowledge in the service of humanity through learning, justice and faith" (Loyola University Chicago, 2010, The Loyola Mission section, para.1). Specifically, this involves being part of a learning community that values self-critical reflection as part of the process of improving the operations of the university and preparing students to lead productive lives. Promoting activities that emphasize reflection illustrates the university's emphasis on transformational learning.

Recommendations

Feedback collected from students revealed several areas in which there was potential for improvement. The first of these suggestions was to make blogging a requirement of the course. Students stated that having increased participation would provide a wider variety of experiences from which they could learn. Students also suggested that the course include topics covered in the reflection papers. Finally, it was suggested that instructors post all entries well in advance of the reflection paper's due dates, as students expressed the interest in working on assignments in advance and would have liked more timely access to entries.

Several students remarked that contributing comments to the blog helped to improve their writing skills and the way they thought about a particular topic. Students stated that they felt that the ability to post their thoughts on the blog allowed them to focus on content rather than worrying about grammatical errors. For future iterations of the course, students encouraged use of the blog for brainstorming or presenting early drafts of papers. The researchers are interested in identifying rubrics for critical thinking and designing future studies to further illustrate the impact of using a blog on critical thinking.

Implications

The application of experiential learning theory provides a framework for the development of critical thinking using current technology. Blogs and other social networking services are rapidly becoming an integral part of our personal, academic, and professional lives. Integration of such technology in an academic course to further pedagogical goals is a positive and progressive mode of encouraging deep learning and critical thinking. This study illustrates the power of the reflective-writing process to promote understanding of one's self and capabilities. Using blog technology encouraged participation and interaction, increased understanding of select subjects, and introduced new ways of learning. Faculty who conducted this study are hopeful that student nurses who are educated to reflect will have a better understanding of their patients—and themselves—as they enter their profession.

ACKNOWLEDGMENT

The authors acknowledge the contribution of Carol Scheidenhelm, PhD, Director of Learning Technology and Assessment, Loyola University Chicago, for her role as consultant to this project.

References

Billings, D. M. (2009). Wikis and blogs: Consider the possibilities for continuing nursing education. *Journal of Continuing Education in Nursing, 40,* 534–535. doi: 10.3928/00220124-20091119-10

Brixey, J. J., & Warren, J. J. (2009). Creating experiential learning activities using Web 2.0 tools and technologies: A case study. In K. Saranto, P. Flatley Brennan, H. Park, M. Tallberg, & A. Ensio (Eds.), *Studies in Health Technology and Informatics,* (Vol. 146, pp. 613–617). Amsterdam, The Netherlands: IOS Press. doi: 10.3233/978-1-60750-024-7-613

Brockbank, A., & McGill, I. (1998). *Facilitating reflective learning in higher education.* New York, NY: Open University Press.

Burke, S., & Oomen-Earley, J. (2008). That's blog worthy: Ten ways to integrate blogging into the health education classroom. *American Journal of Health Education, 39*(6), 362–364.

Collins, A., Brown, J. S., & Newman, S. E. (1989). Cognitive apprenticeship: Teaching the craft of reading, writing and mathematics. In L. B. Resnick (Ed.), *Knowing, learning and instruction: Essays in honor of Robert Glaser* (pp. 453–494). Hillsdale, NJ: Erlbaum.

Hanson, C., Thackeray, R., Barnes, B., Neiger, B., & McIntyre, E. (2008). Integrating Web 2.0 in health education preparation and practice. *American Journal of Health Education, 39*(3), 157–166.

Kolb, A. Y., & Kolb, D. A. (2009). The learning way: Meta-cognitive aspects of experiential learning. *Simulation & Gaming. 40*, 297–327. doi: 10.1177/1046878108325713

Lisko, S. A., & O'Dell, V. (2010). Integration of theory and practice: Experiential learning theory and nursing education. *Nursing Education Perspectives, 31*(2), 106–108.

Loyola University Chicago (2010). *Mission Statement*. Retrieved from www.luc.edu/loyolapromise/mission.shtml

Scheffer, B. K., & Rubenfeld, M. G. (2000). A consensus statement on critical thinking in nursing. *Journal of Nursing Education, 39*, 352–359.

Shaffer, S. C., Lackey, S. P., & Bolling, G. W. (2006). Blogging as a venue for nurse faculty development. *Nursing Education Perspectives, 27*, 126–127.

Strampel, K., & Oliver, R. (2007). Using technology to foster reflection in higher education. Proceedings from *Ascilite 2007, Singapore: ICT—Providing choices for learners and learning, 2–5 December 2007*. Retrieved from www.ascilite.org.au/conferences/singapore07/procs/strampel.pdf

Zeng, X., & Harris, S. T. (2005). Blogging in an online health information technology class. *Perspectives in Health Information Management: An Online Research Journal, 2*(6), 1–18.

19

Learning through Reflective Practice: Student-Led Panel Presentation on Individualized Aging

Deborah P. Copeland, PhD, RN

Nursing education faces a tremendous challenge to provide adequately educated nurses to address the rapidly increasing number of older adults. The Administration on Aging (2010) estimates that the older adult population will comprise 19 percent of the total US population by the year 2030. This generation of older adults will live longer and be better educated and more racially and ethnically diverse than any previous generation, ensuring that their needs will be much different than the elderly of the past (Institute of Medicine [IOM], 2008). This reality requires evidence-based gerontology course content that is offered in all levels of nursing education programs. To meet the need for a competent and culturally sensitive nursing workforce, nurses must be educated to address the unique and often complex health issues that will occur as a result of this demographic shift. The development of a competent and culturally sensitive nursing workforce occurs through carefully designed nursing educational approaches (Souder et al., 2006).

The National League for Nursing (NLN, 2010) developed an educational competencies model that calls for graduates of nursing programs to promote and enhance human flourishing for patients, families, communities, and themselves. One specific approach to addressing the educational competency of human flourishing is through the use of the Advancing Care Excellence for Seniors (ACES) framework, which is designed to guide nursing education and clinical practice (NLN, 2010). Using this structure, the nursing workforce is taught to view the older adult through the lens of individualized aging, complexity, and life transitions. The outcome of such an initiative is the provision of competent, individualized, and humanistic care to older adults (NLN, 2010).

How does this translate into practice? Nursing education must include innovative and varied student experiences that enhance students' competencies in gerontology nursing. This chapter describes the use of reflective practice in the development of a student-led panel presentation on individualized aging within a cultural context.

REFLECTIVE PRACTICE

According to Kolb (1984), it is not the experience itself that the student learns from but rather the reflection on that experience. Kolb's experiential learning theory (1984) uses a holistic viewpoint that encompasses experience, perception, cognition, and behavior. Kolb believed that learning for real understanding requires a sequence—or cycle—of having an experience, reflecting on the experience, forming abstract concepts and generalizations about the experience, and then testing those concepts in new situations (Kolb, 1984). Reflection is particularly useful to learning when working with real-life situations that have no obvious answers (Moon, 1999). Nursing involves many such situations.

The use of reflective practice in nursing education has evolved as a vehicle to enhance student learning and encourage continuous review of nursing practice. However, the act of self-reflection is more than a method of learning. Rather, Ekebergh (2007) purports reflection is a living process that embodies the whole person within his or her lived experience. It is particularly important within the caring sciences, such as nursing, to provide opportunities for students to support and enhance a reflective attitude (Ekebergh, 2007). Self-reflection and the sharing of these reflections can result in a powerful learning experience. Torsvik and Hedlund (2008) found that the use of reflective dialogue enhanced cultural understanding among nursing students representing two cultures through the opportunity to share thoughts about the experience and reflect on their individual value systems and their personal practice of nursing. The use of reflection in the context of the lived experience of students can be a meaningful way to enrich their learning.

CURRICULUM ENHANCEMENT

The associate degree nursing program at Palm Beach State College in Lake Worth, Florida, recently expanded and clarified the specialized gerontology focus within the curriculum. The process culminated in the addition of a three-hour introduction to aging class, a dedicated long-term care clinical rotation with the use of evidence-based assessment tools, a dedicated service learning experience in local senior centers, and the use of evolving case studies in clinical simulation experiences. In response to this focus, the topic of gerontology competency and care was chosen for the school's Nursing Student Association (NSA) Day. This annual educational program for all current nursing students and faculty is planned and hosted by the nursing students each February. The program for the 2010 event included a presentation on the ACES Framework (NLN, 2010) and a student-led panel discussion.

STUDENT-LED PANEL DISCUSSION

The panel discussion was designed to provide an opportunity for nursing students from our ethnically diverse student body to share their perspectives of individualized aging. Nursing students from all four semesters of the program were invited to participate. The five students who volunteered were asked to reflect on their own cultural values, beliefs, and attitudes toward the older adult and on how their culture met the needs of the older adult. Each was then requested to compose a 10-minute individual presentation for the day.

The students who volunteered were ethnically diverse and represented each semester of the program. One student chose to present in her native language, with another student translating what she said into English. The members of the audience appreciated this unique presentation method. The students freely shared their beliefs and attitudes about their culture's views on aging and how the older adult is cared for within their families.

Several of the students contrasted their personal family experience with their long-term care clinical experience. They discussed the value of the older adult within each of their respective cultural communities, and explained that older adults deserved the respect of all family members. The students explained that elders are cared for within the safety of family, and the use of nursing homes was shunned. Each student demonstrated how aging was viewed as a unique process within and across cultural boundaries.

BENEFITS OF THE EXPERIENCE

A student-led panel discussion provided the opportunity for students to state their unique perspectives regarding a focused topic. The student audience listened to their peers rather than just faculty, and the student panelists provided unique perspectives that faculty could not. The reflection that occurred provided rich examples that helped to broaden awareness of how and where older adults live in the community and strengthened the view that each individual experiences aging in a unique manner.

CONCLUSION

In this particular learning activity, students were able to share their personal experiences, reflect on them, and apply them to new situations that they encountered in the nursing program. Such activities support and enhance the reflective attitudes of the students, providing an essential link between theory and practice. The opportunity to develop a student-led presentation enhances student engagement and is a relatively easy learning activity to implement. The approach described in this chapter was used in a large educational event, but can be easily adapted to the classroom.

References

Administration on Aging. (2010). *Aging Statistics*. Retrieved from www.aoa.gov/AoA-Root/Aging_Statistics/index.aspx

Ekebergh, M. (2007). Lifeworld-based reflection and learning: a contribution to the reflective practice in nursing and nursing education. *Reflective Practice, 8,* 331–343. doi: 10:1080/14623940701424835

Institute of Medicine (IOM). (2008). *Retooling for an aging America: Building the health care workforce.* Washington, DC: National Academies Press.

Kolb, D. A. (1984). *Experiential learning: Experience as the source of learning and development.* Englewood Cliffs, NJ: Prentice-Hall.

Moon, J. A. (1999). *Reflection in learning and professional development.* London: Kogan Page.

National League for Nursing (NLN). (2010). Advancing Care Excellence for Seniors (ACES). Retrieved from www.nln.org

National League for Nursing (NLN). (2010). *Outcomes and competencies for graduates of practice/vocational, diploma, associate degree, baccalaureate, master's, practice doctorate, and research doctorate programs in nursing.* New York, NY: Author. Model retrieved from www.nln.org/facultydevelopment/competencies/index.htm

Souder, E., Kagan, S., Hansen, L., Macera, L., Mobily, P., & White, D. (2006). Innovations in geriatric nursing curricula: Experiences from the John A. Hartford Foundation Centers of Geriatric Nursing Excellence. *Nursing Outlook, 54,* 219–222. doi: 10:1016/j.outlook.200.004

Torsvik, M., & Hedlund, M. (2008). Cultural encounters in reflective dialogue about nursing care: a qualitative study. *Journal of Advanced Nursing, 63,* 389–396. doi: 10.1111/j.1365–2648.2008.04723.x

IV

Advancing Education

Section 4 focuses on advancing education. Advancing the educational preparation of nurses is a well-publicized recommendation of the Institute of Medicine's (IOM) 2011 report, *The Future of Nursing: Leading Change, Advancing Health* (IOM, 2011). Advancing education among nurses focuses not just on increasing the number of baccalaureate-prepared nurses but also on doctoral and continuing education. The three recommendations of the *Future of Nursing* report related to education of nurses are:

- *Recommendation 4:* Increase the proportion of nurses with a baccalaureate degree to 80 percent by 2020.

- *Recommendation 5:* Double the number of nurses with a doctorate by 2020.

- *Recommendation 6:* Ensure that nurses engage in lifelong learning.

These recommendations are applicable to all nurses. Therefore, the possible topics related to advancing education are many and varied. In this section, Chapters 20 through 24 consider advancing nursing education from a variety of perspectives, including ensuring the recommendations from the Institute of Medicine are incorporated into baccalaureate education, partnering of a university and hospital to provide an accelerated RN-to-BSN program, preparing graduate students to enter a DNP program, and assisting faculty in developing their writing abilities, a key component for advancing their own education through publishing, as well as expanding the literature base as a fundamental element of the education for all nurses.

Reference

Institute of Medicine. (2011). *The future of nursing: Leading change, advancing health.* Washington, DC: The National Academies Press.

20

A BSN Action Guide for Responding to the 2011 Institute of Medicine Recommendations

Patty M. Orr, EdD, RN
Lisa M. Ciampini, MS

Since the publication of the landmark document by the Institute of Medicine (IOM), *The Future of Nursing: Leading Change, Advancing Health* (2011), baccalaureate of science nursing (BSN) programs have been asking themselves: What changes can be made now to begin implementation of the IOM recommendations? Harvey V. Fineberg, the President of the IOM, states in the *Future of Nursing* foreword:

> This work will serve as a blueprint for how the nursing profession can transform itself into an ever more potent relevant force for lasting solutions to enhance the quality and value of U.S. health care in ways that will meet the future health needs of diverse populations (p. ix).

If the IOM document is to serve as a blueprint for nursing education, nursing programs must develop a plan to begin taking steps to respond to its recommendations.

With the clear IOM goal of advancing the health status of the nation's population, the IOM, in partnership with the Robert Wood Johnson Foundation, encourages nursing education to make profound changes in how future nurses are educated. Baccalaureate nursing education must take responsibility to prepare increased numbers of BSN nurse leaders who can significantly contribute in new roles within the 2014 reformed health care system.

A BSN ACTION GUIDE

The National League for Nursing (NLN) enhanced the magnitude of the IOM publication's potential impact on nursing education's future when the NLN changed its mission statement in February 2011 by adding "to advance the nation's health" to its nursing education philosophy (NLN, 2011). With the support of the IOM and NLN organizations, nursing education programs have the timely opportunity to forge actions to realize execution of the recommendations and impact nursing school graduates' competencies in effectively improving patient health outcomes and the nation's health. This BSN action guide serves as an interpretation of specific actions that can be used by BSN programs;

those actions include an aggressive focus on increasing the numbers of both entry-level and BSN-completion graduates, as well as increasing the number of nurses obtaining a doctoral degree. To assist BSN programs to take action and create their own intervention plan, the following action guide for implementation is proposed. The guide originates from content in *The Future of Nursing* (IOM, 2011), listing specific ideas and action steps for change in response to the recommendations as interpreted from the IOM report. Table 20.1 presents the components of the BSN Action Guide.

With the recommendation to significantly increase the number of nurses with baccalaureate degrees, BSN schools need to increase capacity in entry-level programs and facilitate improved articulation into BSN programs for associate and diploma graduates. Two of the eight IOM recommendations appeal for significant increase in workforce numbers of BSN and doctorally prepared nurses by the year 2020. The IOM asks that 80 percent of RNs hold a BSN degree by 2020. Presently, only 50 percent of the RN workforce has a BSN degree (American Association of Colleges of Nursing [AACN], 2011). BSN program enrollment increased only by 5.7 percent from 2009 to 2010, and no space was available for 57,000 qualified BSN applicants in 2010 (AACN, 2011). To approach the 80 percent mark of BSN graduates, graduation rates need to increase for both entry-level and BSN completion. To accomplish these rates, articulation agreements between nursing education programs need to be in place enabling easy transfer of course credit between community colleges and BSN programs. Currently, 32 states have mandated broad transfer agreements among state nursing programs (AACN, 2011). In other states, many individual agreements are in place between nursing programs within specific community colleges and universities that are in close proximity to each other.

The IOM's request for the aggressive increase in BSN nurses is based on several studies that linked baccalaureate nurses to decreased patient mortality and adverse outcomes (AACN, 2011). In addition, BSN nurses significantly pursue graduate-level education compared to associate degree nurses. Increased numbers of nurses with doctoral degrees are needed to fill the many vacant faculty positions in BSN programs; these vacant positions are a factor that limits admission of qualified applicants.

INCREASING DOCTORALLY PREPARED NURSES

In response to the significant deficit of doctorally prepared nurses, the IOM recommends that the number of nurses with doctoral degrees double by 2020. Doctorally prepared nurses are needed for primary care, advanced practice roles, research, and faculty positions. To attract nurses earlier in their career to doctoral study, 73 BSN-to-PhD programs within 22 states provide an option for direct progression from a BSN degree to a PhD degree (AACN, 2011). These BSN-to-PhD programs are similar to other science-based professions that require doctoral degrees prior to practicing. The rationale is that if nurses are younger when they receive their PhD, they will be able to practice as faculty members or researchers for a longer period of time.

The number of students presently in doctoral programs is increasing, with a 25.6 percent increase in enrollment in DNP programs from 2009 to 2010 and a 4.5 percent growth in PhD and DNSc program enrollment (AACN, 2011). These increases are encouraging; however, the current rate of graduation from doctoral programs indicates potential gaps in the ability to double the number of doctoral graduates by 2020.

TABLE 20.1

BSN School of Nursing Action Guide for Implementing IOM Recommendations

IOM Recommendations	BSN Program Actions
1. Remove scope-of-practice barriers.	1. Transform the utilization of nurses across settings and act as partners in the health care team.[a] 2. Examine innovative solutions related to care delivery by focusing on the delivery of nursing services (e.g., telephonic care calls after hospital discharge).[a] 3. Remove legal and financial barriers (support legislative intervention). 4. Prepare students to help patients prevent and/or manage chronic illnesses, thus preventing exacerbations and disease complications.[a] 5. Facilitate education opportunities in the clinical and classroom setting with physicians and other health professionals (students work with the medical director to download information on all patients with identified indicators of poor health status such as high body mass index [BMI] and project manage call campaigns).[a] 6. Address insufficient clinical placement opportunities and shortage of clinical faculty (consider nurse-managed health centers, dedicated clinical education units [DEUs], partnerships in community health center settings).[a] 7. Practice with nurse practitioners as a team for care of the elderly or other at-risk populations.[a]
2. Expand opportunities for nurses to lead and diffuse collaborative improvement efforts.	1. Prepare students to assume leadership roles and fill new and expanded roles in the redesigned system of health care.[a] 2. Facilitate students' practice in care delivery models in which nurses, physicians, and other health professionals collaborate with effective delivery of care interventions that result in improved patient outcomes.[a] 3. Prepare students to collect and manage nursing-focused quality indicators.[a] 4. Provide opportunities to screen large at-risk populations and provide care intervention for those at risk (market to people at risk for diabetes and high BMI and register them to attend screenings to assess risk with fasting plasma glucose (FPG) assessment).[a] 5. Prepare students to envision and execute systems of care that promote patient health outcome improvement.[a] 6. Prepare students to measure and document the outcomes of their interventions.[a] 7. Teach students to practice as a full partner and collaborate with physicians and other health professionals.[a]

(continued)

TABLE 20.1

BSN School of Nursing Action Guide for Implementing IOM Recommendations (Continued)

IOM Recommendations	BSN Program Actions
3. Implement nurse residency programs.	1. Manage the transition from school to practice; assist and partner in the development of residency programs in acute and nonacute care settings. 2. Develop partnerships with provider organizations.[a] 3. Partner with hospitals to develop DEUs for clinical site assignment, and contribute to the development of residency programs. 4. Consider assisting in development of nonacute residency programs by increasing emphasis on community and public health in the classroom and clinical settings. 5. Increase emphasis placed on developing competencies in community and public health, primary care, geriatrics, disease prevention, and health promotion.[a]
4. Increase the proportion of nurses with a baccalaureate degree to 80 percent by 2020.	1. Recruit and support diverse students with funding and remediation support if needed to complete the program.[a] 2. Provide seamless advancement of students from ADN to BSN by partnering with community colleges and vocational schools.[a] 3. Develop a transferrable curriculum that articulates between state community colleges and universities.[a] 4. Affiliate with associate degree nursing programs in the same geographical part of the state to facilitate in-person marketing and counseling with potential students.[a] 5. Implement technology, such as simulation and electronic health records.[a] 6. Incorporate distance learning with online courses.[a] 7. Market RN-to-BSN programs to RNs, and health organization employers.[a] 8. Prepare students with a skill set to retrieve and manage information and data.[a] 9. Appeal to stakeholders for financial support for faculty doctoral study.[a]
5. Double the number of nurses with a doctorate by 2020.	1. Prepare BSN students for aspiring to achieve MSN and doctoral nursing degrees in order to practice as primary care providers, researchers, and nurse faculty.[a] 2. Prepare students to transition to graduate programs of study after completion of the BSN program curriculum.[a] 3. Require senior students to address their goal for graduate study in their professional portfolio.[a] 4. Encourage a lifelong learner mindset, development of beginning skills as a researcher, and interest in disease prevention for populations.[a] 5. Support MSN faculty with financial and scheduling support to complete doctoral study.[a]

TABLE 20.1

BSN School of Nursing Action Guide for Implementing
IOM Recommendations (Continued)

IOM Recommendations	BSN Program Actions

6. Ensure that nurses engage in lifelong learning.	1. Prepare nurses to practice in an evolving health care system and deliver safe and patient-centric care in community and public health settings.[a]
	2. Include BSN nurse education content and practice in:[a]
	  a. Evidence-based practice
	  b. Research
	  c. Interdisciplinary teamwork performance
	  d. Collaboration and care coordination
	3. Initiate a competency-based approach to education. Course competencies are explicit and entail daily inquiry, systems thinking, care management, and process improvement.[a]
	  a. Increase skills assessment for all faculty and students.
	  b. Include research–based analysis of outcome data assignment in all courses.
	  c. Create a foundation for decision making in varied clinical situations.
	4. Prepare to provide holistic, patient-centered care and respond to social, mental, and spiritual needs.[a]
	5. Teach and practice process and quality improvement initiatives. Identify and measure change metrics and trends.[a]

7. Prepare and enable nurses to lead change to advance health.	1. Teach students to practice to the full extent of their education and training.[a]
	2. Prepare students to envision practice in an evolving health care system; provide practice opportunities in evolving health care systems.[a]
	3. Support inclusion of NCLEX measurement of competencies related to community and public health, geriatrics, health promotion, and disease prevention.
	4. Prepare students for emerging competencies in:[a]
	  a. Decision making
	  b. Quality improvement
	  c. Systems thinking
	  d. Transitional care at hospital discharge
	5. Teach students to embrace continuing and professional education in order to seek opportunities to exercise their leadership skills to help transform the health care system, which leads to effective outcomes for patients.[a]
	6. Teach students to use technological tools to improve quality and effectiveness of care interventions (e.g., electronic health record, simulation, data management, and distance learning).[a]
	7. Teach students to provide safer and more effective care with ethical integrity.[a]

(continued)

TABLE 20.1

BSN School of Nursing Action Guide for Implementing
IOM Recommendations (*Continued*)

IOM Recommendations	BSN Program Actions

	8. Teach students to analyze and develop a systems approach to better care intervention.[a]
	9. Update and adapt curriculum to meet changing health care needs by achieving new competencies to:[a]
	  a. Improve quality and safety goal achievement for patients
	  b. Achieve prevention of disease, promote wellness, and improve health outcome achievement
	  c. Provide effective care coordination
	10. Prepare students to provide nurse-directed holistic care management, transitional care, and coordination of complex care needs.[a]

8. Build an infrastructure for the collection and analysis of interprofessional health care workforce data.	1. Support and participate in all nursing surveys requesting information regarding the health care workforce.[a] 2. Document and track all nursing students upon entry into a nursing program. Collect demographic data, ethnicity, completion status, grades, and employment for all class cohorts, and report as requested for workforce data collection.[a] 3. Provide clinical opportunities for students to practice in teams with other health care professionals.[a] 4. Facilitate racial, ethnic, and gender diversity of the nursing student body and track minority status with a database.[a] 5. Prepare students to lead and innovate in developing patient-centered care models that improve health outcomes and reduce cost.[a] 6. Integrate business practices and leadership theory across the curriculum. Include competencies in health care policy and financing.[a] 7. Collect and manage data related to interprofessional experiences and competencies.[a] 8. Prepare students for data collection and information infrastructure utilization.[a]

[a]Represents program action currently implemented at our school.

Our school is bolstering an increase in doctorally prepared faculty by providing financial assistance to MSN faculty. Faculty members pursuing a doctoral degree are receiving significant tuition reimbursement and clinical release time to attend doctoral programs (either PhD or DNP). Doctorally prepared faculty are needed to prepare increased numbers of BSN graduates, and are also needed to prepare graduates who meet the changing employer expectations for nurses who can intervene consistently to achieve positive patient outcome improvements.

PREPARING BSN STUDENTS FOR EXPANDED ROLES

In addition to increasing BSN student capacity and supporting faculty attainment of doctoral degrees, our school is taking action to lead change and advance health by preparing BSN students for expanded roles that will impact the health status of patients in the community setting. The faculty of the School of Nursing at Austin Peay State University have developed a community health center partnership that provides students an opportunity to create innovation in the delivery of nursing care in a community setting. Students practice as a collaborative team to impact the health status of an underserved population and develop competencies in disease management, health promotion, care coordination, and gerontology. Scalable innovative methods of intervention by BSN students in this setting include the use of telephonic care calls, care card reminders, disease-specific call campaigns, and disease-specific group classes. The experience differs from traditional community health clinical experiences in that students are responsible for delivering nursing actions and held accountable for improving certain health status metrics for a population.

An example of one initiative includes downloading patient information on all patients with an HbA1c greater than 7 percent. These patients receive care calls by the BSN students to determine the patient's success in managing their diabetes. During the care call patients are invited to and scheduled for group classes to help them with medication adherence, blood glucose monitoring, diet, and exercise. BSN students prepare and facilitate the group classes. Reminder cards sent by mail reinforce individual goals set by patients during care calls or in class. Students coordinate care with the provider by tracking and reporting the ongoing HbA1c response to intervention for the patients with whom they intervene. Practice in this nonacute environment exposes students to leadership experience in analyzing patients' response to nursing interventions, and reporting of corresponding outcome data for a population.

PLANNING FOR THE FUTURE

The School of Nursing at Austin Peay State University also provides two learning activities that prepare students for graduate study articulation after BSN completion. All senior students are required to describe their plan for graduate study in their professional portfolios, which are used for employment or further education purposes. Senior students are also required to write a formal ethical dilemma paper. Faculty members, who primarily teach in the MSN program, guide students as they develop their topic and proposal. The ethical dilemma paper serves as a bridge assignment that introduces scholarly writing and synthesis in preparation for graduate study.

CLOSING REMARKS

Each BSN school of nursing must strategize the development of a plan of action with specific tactics for implementing the IOM recommendations. BSN educators have an opportunity to not only increase the numbers of graduates, but to prepare students for lifelong learning and to lead change to advance health. Patients will be the ultimate recipients of positive changes in education, demonstrating improved health outcomes by preventing disease progression and complications. By consistently improving patient outcomes, the nation's health will advance. Each BSN school of nursing must ask: What changes can be made now to the nursing program and how does implementation begin? This action guide puts a tool in the hands of BSN educators that will facilitate their timely action for transforming education.

References

American Association of Colleges of Nursing (AACN). (2011, April 14). Creating a more highly qualified nursing workforce. Retrieved from www.AACN.nche.edu.

Institute of Medicine (IOM). (2011). *The future of nursing: Leading change, advancing health*. Washington, DC: The National Academies Press.

National League for Nursing (NLN). (2011, February 28). National League for Nursing revises mission statement to reflect ongoing focus on nation's health: Agility, responsiveness, and sensitivity mark mission modification and new living documents series. Retrieved from http://www.nln.org/newsreleases/mission_livingdocs_022811.htm.

21

A Hospital-Based, University-Run, Cohort Hybrid Model:
RN-to-BSN Degree

Kerry A. Milner, DNSc, RN

The Institute of Medicine (IOM) report, *The Future of Nursing: Leading Change, Advancing Health* (2011) report calls for 80 percent of nurses to hold a BSN degree by 2020. To achieve this, working RNs must have access to flexible and innovative BSN programs that work best for them personally, professionally, and financially. A recent national survey of RN-to-BSN programs revealed the published literature lacking in information specific to these programs (McEwen, White, Pullis, & Krawtz, 2012). Survey results indicate that most nursing program settings are in universities (92 percent) and not hospitals (4 percent).

An intensive search of the literature of the last 5 years using CINAHL, MEDLINE, Academic Search Premier, and ERIC databases was conducted using keywords *RN to BSN, hybrid,* and/or *blended learning.* No articles described a hospital-based, university-run, cohort hybrid RN-to-BSN model with classes meeting at the hospital. Davidson, Metzger, & Lindgren (2011) described a successful university-run cohort hybrid model with classes held at the university.

This chapter describes an innovative hospital-based, university-run hybrid accelerated RN-to-BSN program that is educating nurses at their workplace and achieving the goal of creating an educational environment in which the postlicensure student can succeed.

ADVANTAGES OF A SMALL ONSITE COHORT

Some hospitals offer incentives to influence enrollment in a BSN program; offering classes at the workplace is a top-ranking incentive (Warren & Mills, 2009). Onsite classes offer easy accessibility to RNs returning for a BSN, as such students have many competing obligations. A small onsite cohort encourages peer collaboration, support, and continued motivation to complete the program. The workplace class model provides direct social contact with peers and faculty, which can decrease feelings of anxiety and isolation for the adult learner returning to school (Davidson, Metzger, & Lindgren, 2011).

ADVANTAGES OF HYBRID LEARNING

A hybrid course design can use 50 percent face-to-face teaching and 50 percent online instruction. Hybrid design gives the adult learner desired flexibility and a sense of control over the timing of the learning (Davidson, Metzger, & Lindgren, 2011). Busy RNs are more apt to seek an advanced degree when the course delivery is a mix of flexible online and traditional instruction (Megginson, 2008; Teeley, 2007). A hybrid design can be multisensory, meeting the needs of a variety of learning styles, and has been shown to be an effective strategy for educating nurses (Ireland et al., 2009; McCain, 2008).

The advantages of using a hybrid model include new teaching opportunities, increased student engagement and learning, and new pedagogical approaches. The hybrid model allows faculty to develop and use a variety of online and in-class teaching strategies to meet course objectives. Faculty use new types of interactive and independent learning activities that are not possible in purely online or purely traditional face-to-face RN-to-BSN courses. This pedagogical approach has been associated with high levels of satisfaction in Taiwanese nursing students in RN-to-BSN programs (Hsu, 2011) and in practicing nurses in the United States (Smith & Gordon, 2009).

Faculty–student and student–student connectivity is one attribute of a hybrid course that is especially helpful. For example, there can be fluidity with online and face-to-face discussions. Integration of the traditional and online formats allows for faculty to make more effective use of class time. In a successful hybrid environment, a variety of participatory and student-centered learning activities are used. The faculty role changes from "sage on the stage" to a learner-centered facilitator, or "guide on the side." Pedagogical efficiency can be increased when faculty use online time to automate basic activities such as quizzes, grading, and surveys (De George-Walker & Keeffe, 2010). Additionally, online documentation of group work increases ease of student assessments. Lastly, the hybrid format works well with the student's work schedules. Nurses are able to feel connected with face-to-face sessions meeting at their workplace, then complete the work for the online portion around their work and family schedules.

There is a dearth of published research examining the learning outcomes of RN-to-BSN nursing students who take courses in a hybrid environment. Hsu & Hsieh (2011) reported an increase in metacognitive and self-regulatory development in Taiwanese RN-to-BSN students enrolled in a hybrid professional nursing ethics course. These authors also noted that the increased metacognitive skills developed in a hybrid course improved the nursing student's ability to solve tough clinical problems. More research needs to be done comparing learning outcomes in strictly online courses with hybrid courses.

HYBRID LEARNING CHALLENGES

Successful hybrid course design is not simply a transfer of a portion of a traditional BSN course to the online environment. It can be challenging for faculty to examine their course goals and objectives of the traditional BSN courses and decide which are best taught as an online learning activity and which need to be taught in a classroom. It can be difficult to successfully integrate online and classroom learning components. A pitfall of hybrid design can be assigning too many online activities or covering too much material, resulting in content overload. For some faculty, it may be difficult to transition from a lecture method to a student-centered active learning approach. Traditional methods for student assessment may not be effective in the hybrid environment. Faculty may need assistance learning on how to facilitate online discussions and small group activities as well as planning appropriate assessment methods (Glogowska, Young, Lockyer, & Moule, 2011; Ransdell & Gaillard-Kenney, 2009).

The hybrid environment requires different types of learning supports. The hybrid environment adds additional scheduling and communication challenges because courses meet both online and face to face. A hybrid, accelerated RN-to-BSN program can be challenging for RNs as they adjust to the use of technology and to the fast pace of these courses (Glogowska, Young, Lockyer, & Moule, 2011). Students may require a significant amount of support as they adapt to an active learner role, to the new technology, and to management of online and classroom work. Faculty must also consider personal characteristics of the learner when designing and implementing a hybrid course (Hsu & Hsieh, 2011). For example, students who graduated more than 15 years ago may not have the computer and web-based skills needed to navigate the online learning environment and may benefit from a structured face-to-face orientation to the online platform and other university technology requirements.

HOSPITAL-BASED, UNIVERSITY-RUN, ONSITE COHORT HYBRID MODEL

The program described in this chapter provides an opportunity for RNs employed in the same hospital to complete 62 credits in two calendar years to fulfill the requirements for a BSN. Classes are scheduled as eight-week sessions, with nursing courses offered in a hybrid design and nonnursing courses offered online (see Table 21.1). In consideration of personal needs, time off from classes is scheduled during the holiday periods and in the summer. The cohort portion of this program consists of a class of qualified students who start and continue through the program as a group. This approach is associated with higher degree completion and satisfaction rates (Davidson, Metzger, & Lindgren, 2011). Admission criteria include an active RN license, employment at the sponsoring hospital, and a prelicense nursing program grade point average of greater than 2.5.

INFRASTRUCTURE TO SUPPORT THE PROGRAM

A successful onsite cohort hybrid program needs strong leadership and an established infrastructure to meet program needs. Presently, this program is offered at four hospitals under the supervision of a director who has an active RN license and MSN degree with extensive experience teaching in BSN and MSN programs. She has leadership experience as a vice president of nursing for a small hospital for 12 years and has held several clinical positions. The director and faculty were hired exclusively for this program; faculty who teach in the program hold an MSN degree. The majority of the nursing courses are taught by full-time faculty; fewer than 25 percent are taught by adjunct faculty.

TABLE 21.1

Curriculum Sequence: Hospital-Based, University-Run, Onsite Cohort Hybrid Model Course

Year 1	Year 2
August–October **Transition to Professional Practice** The Art of Thinking	*September–October* **Evidence-Based Practice** The Individual and Society
October–December **Information Technology for Nursing Practice** Literary Expressions of the Human Journey	*October–December* **Leadership in Contemporary Nursing Practice** Introduction to the Study of Religion
January–March The Human Journey: Historical Paths to Civilization Math for Health Professions	*January–March* Bioethics: Religious Approaches The Human Search for Truth, Justice and the Common Good
March–May **The Human Journey in Nursing** Statistics for Decision Making	*March–May* **Care Management: Individuals and Families** Humanities Elective
May–July **Health Assessment for RNs** Introduction to Problems of Philosophy	*May–July* **Public and Global Health** Humanities Elective

Hybrid nursing courses are in bold.

The hospitals and university work collaboratively to recruit qualified RNs. The hospital recruiter, along with the program director, schedules onsite information sessions for interested nurses. Potential students submit an application to the university and the director conducts onsite interviews. Students who meet all criteria are admitted on a first-come, first-served basis until all 25 spots are filled.

Support from the hospitals includes an attractive financial package to assist students with tuition and priority work schedules built around class times. The two-year curriculum sequence was designed to work with the scheduling parameters of the hospitals. The hospitals provide the necessary audiovisual equipment, classroom space, and technology support such as electronic whiteboards and Internet access. The university provides online and technical support as well as individual training when needed. Using Blackboard© as the online course management system, faculty adopted a standardized menu format for announcements, syllabi, information, and

TABLE 21.2

Demographic Characteristics of the Six Cohorts (N = 69)

Characteristic	Mean or Percent
Mean age (years)[a]	42
Gender	
Female	97 percent
Male	3 percent
Race[b]	
White	74 percent
African American	20 percent
Hispanic	6 percent
Overall graduation rate	80 percent

[a]missing n = 28
[b]missing n = 5

discussions. A face-to-face orientation on navigation of the online platform is part of the first course.

STUDENT CHARACTERISTICS

Six cohorts have successfully graduated between 2001 and 2011 with an average graduation rate of 80 percent (86 total admissions and 69 graduates). Students who left the program did so primarily because of a change in job or life circumstances. Some students who changed jobs transferred to the online or traditional program and completed their BSN (n = 6). Therefore, the actual average BSN graduation rate was higher. Only one student was asked to leave the program because of course failure. Demographic characteristics of those who graduated are presented in Table 21.2. Students were predominantly white females with a mean age of 42 years, ranging from 27 to 64 years of age.

CONCLUSION

This hospital-based, university-run, onsite cohort hybrid model is an innovative and highly successful way for nurse educators to efficiently increase the education level of the RN workforce while maintaining quality and satisfaction. This model has met the educational as well as social needs for working professional nurses as evidenced by an 80 percent graduation rate over 10 years. The onsite, cohort, hybrid combination maximizes connectedness with flexibility to address the needs of employed RNs to earn a BSN degree.

References

Davidson, S. C., Metzger, R., & Lindgren, K. S. (2011). A hybrid classroom-online curriculum format for RN-BSN students: Cohort support and curriculum structure improve graduation rates. *Journal of Continuing Education in Nursing, 42*(5), 223–232.

De George-Walker, L. & Keeffe, M. (2010). Self-determined blended learning: A case study of blended learning design. *Higher Education Research and Development, 29*(1), 1–13.

Glogowska, M., Young, P., Lockyer, L., & Moule, P. (2011). How 'blended' is blended learning?: Students' perceptions of issues around the integration of online and face-to-face learning in a continuing professional development (CPD) health care context. *Nurse Education Today, 31*, 887–891.

Hsu, L. (2011). Blended learning in ethics education: A survey of nursing students. *Nursing Ethics, 18*(3), 418–430.

Hsu, L., & Hsieh, S. (2011). Factors associated with learning outcome of BSN in a blended learning environment. *Contemporary Nurse: A Journal for the Australian Nursing Profession, 38*(1/2), 24–34.

Institute of Medicine (IOM). (2011). *The future of nursing: Leading change, advancing health.* Washington, DC: The National Academies Press.

Ireland, J., Martindale, S., Johnson, N., Adams, D., Eboh, W., & Mowatt, E. (2009). Blended learning in education: Effects on knowledge and attitude. *British Journal of Nursing, 18*(2), 124–130.

McCain, C.L. (2008). The right mix to support electronic medical record training classroom computer based training and blended learning. *Journal for Nursing in Staff Development, 24*(4), 151–154.

McEwen, M., White, M., Pullis, B., & Krawtz, S. (2012). National survey of RN-to-BSN programs. *Journal of Nursing Education, 51*(7), 373–380.

Megginson, L. A. (2008). RN-BSN education: 21st century barriers and incentives. *Journal of Nursing Management, 16*(1), 47–55.

Ransdell, S. & Gaillard-Kenney, S. (2009). Blended learning environments, active participation, and student success. *Internet Journal of Allied Health Sciences & Practice, 7*(1), 1–4.

Smith, T., & Gordon, T. (2009). Developing spiritual and religious care competencies in practice: Pilot of a Marie Curie blended learning event. *International Journal of Palliative Nursing, 15*(2), 86–92.

Teeley, K. (2007). Designing hybrid web-based courses for accelerated nursing students. *Journal of Nursing Education, 46*(9), 417–422.

Warren, J., & Mills, M. (2009). Motivating registered nurses to return for an advanced degree. *Journal of Continuing Education in Nursing, 40*(5), 200–207.

22

Preparing MSN Students for Entry into a DNP Program

Karen J. Polvado, DNP, RN, FNP-BC

The doctor of nursing practice (DNP) degree reflects a major transition in doctoral nursing education. The DNP provides a choice for nurses who want to pursue a doctorate with a focus on clinical nursing practice rather than the traditional research-focused PhD degree. The value of the DNP for nursing practice and health care outcomes is not yet known, but its popularity is evident, with more than a 26 percent increase in enrollment between 2008 and 2009 (American Association of Colleges of Nursing [AACN], 2011). This increase in enrollment is possible due to an astonishing increase in DNP programs in the United States. In the spring of 2005, eight DNP programs were offered nationwide. In 2010, the number of DNP programs surpassed the number of research-focused (PhD) programs (153 to 124, respectively; AACN, 2011). In addition, more than 100 schools are considering starting a DNP program. This shift toward the clinical or practice doctorate was an expected evolutionary change in nursing education in response to changes in the health care environment (Chism, 2010).

The Institute of Medicine's (IOM) report, *The Future of Nursing: Leading Change, Advancing Health,* calls for a more highly-educated nursing workforce to deal with a complex, layered health care system (IOM, 2011). According to the National Organization for Nurse Practitioner Faculties (NONPF, 2005), the DNP is needed to prepare nurses to practice in complex health care systems and, as such, should be the terminal degree for advanced practice nursing (APN). Regardless of which organization is advocating for the shift to the practice doctorate, nurses need to level the playing field in terms of status between nurses and other doctorally prepared health care providers such as pharmacists, physical therapists, occupational therapists, and psychologists. Equal status among colleagues can strengthen interprofessional relationships and collaborations (Kaplan & Brown, 2009).

THE PRACTICE DOCTORATE

Practice- and research-focused doctoral programs in nursing share rigorous and demanding expectations. Both degrees are considered terminal degrees in the discipline of nursing; however, there are some distinct differences. Practice-focused programs place greater emphasis on practice and usually include clinical experiences, culminating with the implementation of a practice-oriented final DNP project (AACN, 2006). Research-focused programs focus on the generation of new knowledge and involve a research study. As such, practice-focused, or DNP, programs may better prepare graduates for APN roles.

DNP programs in the United States offer a variety of APN track options, from nurse practitioner to nursing leadership. However, the typical DNP or PhD curriculum does not prepare the graduate for a faculty teaching role (Chism, 2010). Graduates who plan to teach require preparation in teaching methodologies, pedagogical theory, and program evaluation. Some DNP and PhD programs offer an education cognate to prepare the graduate for a faculty teaching role. In addition, some DNP programs are initially offered to in-house faculty who want to pursue a doctorate and to fulfill the need for qualified DNP-prepared faculty at their institutions.

Currently, the primary educational pathway for the DNP is the post-master's degree (Kaplan & Brown, 2009). The demand to increase the number of nurses with advanced degrees will result in a more seamless pathway from post-baccalaureate degree to DNP than is currently in place; but this shift to the post-baccalaureate pathway will take time. In the meantime, many masters in nursing (MSN) programs continue and many of their graduates will pursue doctoral education. Therefore, MSN programs should consider preparing their graduates for a practice-focused doctoral education.

PREPARATION FOR THE PRACTICE DOCTORATE

MSN programs were once considered a predoctorate or mini-PhD program. The master thesis was designed to prepare the student for doctoral education, specifically research-focused doctoral education. However, not all MSN programs require a thesis. Students are often given a choice of thesis or nonthesis as a graduate capstone option. The nonthesis option usually consists of a formal written paper and/or an oral comprehensive examination. Nonthesis options are common for the once-considered terminal degree programs such as nurse practitioner programs. In fact, the nonthesis option was often advised for students with no interest in pursuing a research doctorate.

Prior to 2009, students pursuing an MSN (nurse practitioner, nurse educator, or nurse administrator options) at Midwestern State University, Wilson School of Nursing had two capstone options: thesis or nonthesis. The thesis option consisted of two courses, Thesis I and Thesis II, each worth three semester credit hours (SCH). The Thesis I course was devoted to prospectus development and proposal presentation, while Thesis II involved study implementation, measurement, and analysis. The nonthesis option consisted of two courses, Research Paper I and Research Paper II, each worth three SCH. The research paper courses involved the implementation of a petit project and final paper. The Research Paper I course was devoted to developing a prospectus, while Research Paper II involved implementation and evaluation of a project.

Course evaluations by students and faculty revealed problems with both capstone options. Students often struggled with the steps required to complete a thesis because, in part, they were striving to be clinicians, educators, and administrators, not researchers. The research-paper option was equally difficult because the student was required to implement and evaluate a project. A student in either option was required to select a faculty chairperson and a graduate advisory committee, preferably all with an interest and/or level of expertise in the student's topic. The design and scope of the projects varied and lacked consistency because of the individual differences and levels of preparation of the faculty. Students had difficulty selecting an appropriate topic and often took more than three semesters to complete the work. In addition, our nursing program had a limited number of faculty who were qualified to direct theses, and for those who were, the compensation did not match the amount of time required. There were no hours counting as workload for faculty who directed research papers—it was an expectation of graduate faculty. These factors, combined with the shift toward and popularity of DNP programs, created an environment ready for change. According to the National League for Nursing (NLN, 2004), excellence in nursing education requires a flexible, adaptive curriculum that is responsive to current health care trends and issues. Therefore, a decision was made to replace our current nonthesis option with an evidence-based project series.

THE EVIDENCE-BASED PROJECT SERIES

The evidence-based project (EBP) series was developed to create a more meaningful and comprehensive capstone experience for graduate nursing students. According to the NLN, a hallmark of excellence in nursing education includes a curriculum that ensures that "the curriculum provides learning experiences that prepare graduates to assume roles that are essential to quality nursing practice, including but not limited to those of care provider, patient advocate, teacher, communicator, change agent, care coordinator, user of information, technology, collaborator and decision maker" (Adams & Valiga, 2009, p. 47). The focus of the EBP series is on the development, implementation, and evaluation of an EBP, a project that translates evidence into a change in a health care setting. The logic model—a project planning model—is the framework used to guide students through the phases of project planning. Students learn how to develop project outcomes, objectives, and activities; scan the environment in which the change is to occur; identify stakeholders; create a project budget and marketing plan; implement the project; and evaluate the project. The central tenet of the EBP series is the translation of current and relevant research to the practice setting.

The EBP series and thesis options are equally demanding and have similar learning outcomes that demonstrate synthesis of information at the graduate level. For example, students in both thesis and nonthesis (EBP) options:

- Select topics of interest with a connection to nursing
- Perform an in-depth review and synthesis of relevant literature
- Demonstrate effective communication—both oral and written

In contrast, students in the EBP option plan, implement, and evaluate a project, whereas students in the thesis option plan, implement, and analyze a research study.

MSN-prepared nurses should be ready to assume the role of change agent. The EBP curriculum was designed to provide the graduate student with the knowledge, skills, and abilities to create and foster evidence-based change in a variety of health care settings from acute in-patient hospital settings to rural primary health care settings. In addition, the EBP curriculum was designed to prepare the graduate student for practice-focused doctoral education.

THE CURRICULUM

The objectives of the EBP series are congruent with outcomes for MSN programs. As such, the series is an appropriate nonthesis option for graduate nursing students in our nurse practitioner, nurse educator, and nurse administrator degree options. The course content is innovative and integrates evidence-based nursing education. Students enrolled in the EBP series receive didactic instruction on project planning from qualified and experienced faculty. The students move through the series in a cohort and are given opportunities to develop peer critiquing and senior leadership skills. Successful completion of the EBP series includes a formal comprehensive paper detailing the project and a formal presentation to graduate nursing students and faculty.

The EBP series consists of three courses, each worth two SCH, for a total of six SCH. The EBP courses must be taken sequentially and the students matriculate through the series with a cohort. The course faculty must be doctorally prepared, preferably DNP, but can be PhD prepared with experience in project design, implementation, and evaluation. A maximum is a set of 10 students per cohort per faculty. The series is integrated with specific outputs expected at the completion of each course.

Evidence-Based Project I (EBP I)

The outputs for EBP I include a problem statement and rationale, project objectives, and an executive summary. Students are expected to identify a project champion or mentor at the end of the first EBP course, preferably a person of power and/or influence in the project setting. The students are introduced to peer critiquing, which is a common concept throughout the series.

Evidence-Based Project II (EBP II)

The outputs for EBP II include a draft written paper, an oral presentation of the project proposal, and a project evaluation plan. The paper includes project activities with a timeline, market analysis, strengths-weaknesses-opportunities-threats (SWOT) analysis, and project budget. The students are expected to implement their projects at the end of EBP II.

Evidence-Based Project III (EBP III)

The outputs for EBP III include a final written paper and an oral presentation of the project. The students continue with implementation and evaluation of their projects throughout the last course in the EBP series. Peer critiquing continues and is weighted to reflect increased competence in providing meaningful critique.

THE PROJECTS

Students who completed the first EBP series designed, implemented, and evaluated a wide variety of projects. Two students implemented patient safety goals in a clinical setting (communication, fall prevention). Another student developed a rapid-response team for acute inpatient stroke, while another student instituted policy change to reduce the risk of community-acquired methicillin-resistant *Staphylococcus aureus* (CA-MRSA) in college athletes. One student developed a patient-education program for heart failure and another student implemented a metabolic syndrome screening protocol for a primary health care clinic. The diversity of the projects is a reflection of the individuality of the students and the collegial dialogue and interaction among faculty and students.

CONCLUSION

The first cohort completed the EBP series in the spring of 2010 and provided valuable feedback. In general, the students had difficulty with the logic model format, specifically with the terminology and the concept of backward design. Students also had difficulty narrowing the scope of their projects to a manageable size. Lack of stakeholder involvement early in project planning created some feasibility problems for some students. The students also experienced difficulty giving meaningful peer critique, especially in the first course of the series. Finally, the students reported that more time was needed for project implementation.

In response to feedback from students and faculty, the EBP courses were revised. Following the revision, more time and emphasis were placed on project scope, logic model terminology, and project mentor/champion in the first EBP course. Peer-critiquing learning activities was structured and guided with faculty feedback. Finally, the draft evaluation plan exercise was moved from the beginning of EBP III to the end of EBP II. This move provided the students with more time for project implementation.

Administratively, the EBP series requires less faculty resources than the current thesis or previous research paper options. In the previous nonthesis option, one student project/paper required three graduate faculty committee members: one chairperson and two additional faculty members. In contrast, each EBP course section includes one faculty per 10 graduate students. This assignment requires no additional workload, and faculty commit to following the cohort through the series to completion.

In conclusion, the EBP series prepares the graduate student for advanced practice in a variety of health care settings. This series better prepares the student for doctoral education, specifically the DNP, than the previous approach. The capstone for most DNP programs is a project; therefore, providing the student with the knowledge, skills, and abilities to plan, implement, and evaluate a project will help the student to transition into a DNP program. It is important that APNs (MSN and DNP prepared) possess the skills needed to create and foster change in nursing practice and health care delivery.

References

Adams, M. H., & Valiga, T. M. (2009). *Achieving excellence in nursing education.* New York: National League for Nursing.

American Association of Colleges of Nursing (AACN). (2006, October). *The essentials of doctoral education for advanced nursing practice.* Retrieved from www.aacn.nche.edu/dnp/pdf/essentials.pdf

American Association of Colleges of Nursing (AACN). (2011, March/April). Despite economic challenges, new AACN data confirm sizable growth in doctoral programs. *Syllabus, 37*(2). Retrieved from www.aacn.nche.edu/publications/Syllabus/2011/MarApr11.pdf

Chism, L. A. (2010). *The doctor of nursing practice: A guidebook for role development and professional issues.* Sudbury, MA: Jones & Bartlett.

Institute of Medicine. (2011). *The future of nursing: Leading change, advancing health.* Washington, DC: The National Academies Press. Retrieved from www.iom.edu/Reports/2010/The-Future-of-Nursing-Leading-Change-Advancing-Health.aspx

Kaplan, L., & Brown, M. (2009). Doctor of nursing practice program evaluation and beyond: Capturing the profession's transition to the DNP. *Nursing Education Perspectives, 30*(6), 362–366.

National Organization of Nurse Practitioner Faculties (NONPF). (2005). NONPF recommendations for the nursing practice doctorate and nurse practitioner preparation. Retrieved from www.nonpf.com/associations/10789/files/recommendationsstatement1105.pdf

23

Mentoring Faculty to Write for Publication

Richard L. Pullen, Jr., EdD, RN, CMSRN

Lyndi C. Shadbolt, MS, RN

Advancing the education of nurses is a multifaceted task. One aspect is the issue of advancing the education of nurses providing direct patient care. Another aspect focuses on advancing the educational level of faculty to earn advanced degrees. Faculty also serve as role models for students, supporting the value of advanced degrees.

For any degree, the ability to write is imperative. The need for excellent writing skills is even more intense for graduate-level work; those with advanced degrees represent the most likely group to publish to advance the knowledge base for nursing practice and nursing education. Writing for publication is an essential skill that nursing faculty possess, enabling them to contribute to the body of knowledge in nursing science, enhance patient-centered care, promote professional growth, and gain personal satisfaction. Many nursing faculty who would like to establish a record of publication may fear that their ideas and manuscripts will be rejected, especially those faculty who have little to no writing experience. This chapter presents a mentoring process that helps faculty in a community college nursing department transcend the barriers to writing for publication.

THE VALUE OF PUBLICATION

Writing for peer-reviewed publications is an important professional development strategy. Faculty are encouraged to prepare manuscripts related to research, evidence-based practice (EBP), clinical topics, case studies, innovative teaching strategies, curriculum models and issues impacting nursing, nursing education, and health care (Oermann & Hays, 2011). Faculty can integrate their published works into the teaching and learning experiences for students in the classroom and clinical setting, which supports the scholarship of teaching and application (American Association of Colleges of Nursing [AACN], 2012).

The dissemination of publications in print and electronically is also a way for faculty to teach beyond the walls of their college or university and around the world. Faculty gain personal satisfaction when their published works ultimately enhance the quality of patient care. They are also excited when they see their name in print for the first time.

Barriers to writing for publication are common. Many faculty fear rejection by the editors and may not understand the processes of professional writing (Happell, 2008; Moos & Hawkins, 2009; Oermann & Hays, 2011). Experienced published authors have unique opportunities to serve as mentors for faculty interested in writing for publication.

ESTABLISHING A MENTORSHIP CONNECTION

The value of mentorship in writing for publication became a reality when the primary author (PA) attended a Sigma Theta Tau International (STTI) Honor Society of Nursing Conference in 1997. The PA wanted to learn the "secret" of being published after having a series of manuscripts rejected by editors of peer-reviewed nursing journals. He met a well-noted and esteemed leader in nursing and nursing education at the conference who provided some words of encouragement about the processes of writing for publication. A mentorship connection was established at that moment and has continued throughout the years, primarily through email correspondence. The mentor has a friendly demeanor, a good sense of humor, is an expert in writing for publication and evidence-based nursing practice and education, uses a direct approach when providing guidance, and inspires confidence and creativity in the writing abilities of others. Mentoring relationships promote scholarly productivity, creative expression, and professional growth in nursing (Heinrich & Oberleitner, 2012; McCloughen, O'Brien, & Jackson, 2009). After a series of successful publications, the PA decided to mentor faculty colleagues who expressed an interest in writing for publication.

DEVELOPING A NETWORK OF FACULTY WRITERS

A mentoring process of writing for publication was introduced into the nursing department at Amarillo College in 2001. The purpose of the mentoring process is to help faculty celebrate their ideas, "think outside of the box," inspire confidence, transcend the barriers to writing for publication, promote professional development, and achieve tenure and professorial rank.

Faculty members who desire to write for publication are invited to an annual meeting. A list of topics for writing is generated through a brainstorming session and submitted to the editors of various nursing journals. A detailed outline accompanies each topic. Sometimes editors will initiate contact with faculty in the nursing department to determine if they are interested in writing on a topic for a journal. A subsequent meeting is held when the topics have been approved by journal editors. Roles and responsibilities of the corresponding and primary author and any coauthors are delineated for each manuscript, including a discussion of the criteria for authorship. Timelines are discussed and adhered to as manuscript drafts are reviewed until the final version is submitted electronically to a journal. Consistent guidance and encouragement are part of the mentoring process during the arduous task of manuscript preparation.

FACULTY AND STUDENT OUTCOMES

Since 2001, over 100 publications have appeared in the literature from the Amarillo College nursing department in 15 different peer-reviewed sources. A total of 30 individual faculty members have been the sole author or a coauthor for these publications. Additionally, three nursing faculty from a university setting, three community nurses, one nuclear medicine technology faculty member, and one physician have served as coauthors with the nursing department faculty. A senior-level nursing student was mentored as a coauthor with a faculty member in a recent article. The majority of publications primarily focus on clinical topics that help the nurse to care for a patient; others speak to curriculum models and innovations in nursing education. Publications are indexed in various databases including the Cumulative Index of Nursing and Allied Health Literature (CINAHL), Ovid, International Nursing Index, MEDLINE, Hospital Literature Index, and Current Index to Journals in Education.

Comments from faculty authors about their positive writing experiences include:

- "I can't believe the amount of research I did to prepare the first draft."
- "I am finally published after 20 years as a faculty member."
- "I am using the information in my most recent article to revise didactic instruction."
- "I got a call the other day from a faculty member on the East Coast asking about our published Care Group Model."
- "I have made it a goal to prepare a manuscript at least every six months."
- "The tenure committee was impressed that I had several publications."
- "I would like to be the primary author at some point."

One faculty member stated, "The nursing director where I have clinical rotations with my students posted my article on the bulletin board in the conference room for the nursing staff to use." Published curriculum models have been presented at local, state, and national conferences by the nursing faculty.

Students in the nursing department sometimes cite the literature from the faculty publications when they prepare formal papers in the clinical setting that require critical thinking and clinical reasoning. Students are delighted and even amazed when they locate an article that was published by their nursing instructor(s). Comments from students attest to the positive influence that faculty publications have on their learning:

- "I can't believe that so many of my teachers have published articles."
- "It's nice to know that our instructors help to keep the program up to date with their publications."
- "It's good to know that our instructors have to write formal papers, too."
- "I was able to use two of my instructor's articles when I did my clinical synthesis paper on a patient with cirrhosis of the liver."

It is important for students to realize that their faculty are scholars who want to add to the body of knowledge in evidence-based nursing education and clinical practice through writing projects and other professional activities. Students are encouraged to write for publication as they gain experience in clinical practice and advanced education in nursing. The faculty inspire and mentor students to be the scholars of the future and prepare them to practice nursing in an interprofessional health care world.

References

American Association of Colleges of Nursing (AACN). (2012). Defining scholarship for the discipline of nursing. Retrieved from www.aacn.nche.edu/publications/position/defining-scholarship.

Happell, B. (2008). Writing for publication: A practical guide. *Nursing Standard, 22*(28), 35–40.

Heinrich, K. T., & Oberleitner, M. G. (2012). How a faculty group's mentoring of each other's scholarship can enhance retention and recruitment. *Journal of Professional Nursing, 28*(1), 5–12.

McCloughen, A., O'Brien, L., & Jackson, D. (2009). Esteemed connection: Creating a mentoring relationship for nurse leadership. *Nursing Inquiry, 16*(4), 326–336.

Moos, D. D., & Hawkins, P. H. (2009). Barriers and strategies to the revision process from an editor's perspective. *Nursing Forum, 44*(2), 79–92.

Oermann, M. H., & Hays, J. C. (2011). *Writing for publication in nursing* (2nd ed.). New York, NY: Springer.

24

Promoting Faculty Development through Writing Groups in Online Universities

Deborah S. Adelman, PhD, RN, NE-BC
Alice Raymond, PhD, RN-BC
Timothy J. Legg, PhD, RN-BC, CRNP, GNP-BC, CNE

One aspect of faculty professional development and, often, tenure and promotion, relates to faculty publications in peer-reviewed journals (Peterson & Umphred, 2004). Through writing groups, senior faculty can mentor new and unpublished faculty while encouraging the professional growth of all involved in the process. When faculty teach for online universities, the difficulties associated with formation of writing groups increases. This chapter describes how successful writing groups were created at an online university, Kaplan University, resulting in several publications and articles in press while fostering new research at the university.

LITERATURE REVIEW

Through online collaboration, professionals can overcome limitations imposed by variations in geography, time zones, and language barriers. It is commonplace for colleagues who are separated geographically to coauthor articles. The importance of managing collaboration, laying down principles related to document management, building teams, and attending synchronous and asynchronous meetings are well described in the literature (Kittle & Hicks, 2009; McGrady, 2010; Murphy, Cifuentes, & Shih, 2004; Noël & Robert, 2003; Staggers, Garcia, & Nagelhout, 2008). However, collaboration in writing is more than dividing the tasks of writing and cobbling together a paper. Meaningful collaboration involves each member of the writing group sharing total responsibility for the entire manuscript.

The role of collaboration goes beyond "simply getting along and writing one part" (Kittle & Hicks, 2009, p. 527). However, translating face-to-face techniques for peer-to-peer collaboration presents many challenges when using online communication (Murphy, Cifuentes, & Shih, 2004; Ritchie & Rigano, 2007; Staggers, Garcia, & Nagelhout, 2008). Pivotal to online collaboration is technological literacy, which can positively or adversely affect not only the writing and revising process, but the interpersonal relationships and dynamics of the members of the writing group (McGrady, 2010).

NEW LEADERSHIP, NEW APPROACHES

At a major online university, two faculty members were selected to serve as interim department chairs in the college's BSN and MSN programs. As a component of faculty professional development, these new directors established a six-month goal of initiating faculty-writing groups. The purpose of these groups was consistent with the established literature in that they sought to foster collegiality among full- and part-time faculty, encourage scholarship, and improve teaching in multiple areas consistent with the faculty members' research and practice areas (Kittle & Hicks, 2009; McGrady, 2010; Murphy, Cifuentes, & Shih, 2004; Noël & Robert, 2003; Staggers, Garcia, & Nagelhout, 2008).

The approach used to establish the writing groups was both deliberate and flexible. The approach was deliberate in that establishing the group was the ultimate goal of the endeavor; yet, the approach was flexible because of the multiple competing life demands of the faculty and the desire to accommodate the needs of both full- and part-time faculty.

ASSESSING INTEREST

Once the decision to initiate writing groups was made, the first step in the process involved an assessment of interest in participation among faculty members of the university. The chair of the MSN program emailed all school of nursing faculty. The email explained goals of the writing group and asked if any faculty were interested in participating. Responses poured in from both BSN and MSN faculty; however, not all responses were expected.

Perhaps the most challenging aspect of the endeavor was the wide range of behaviors that emerged. Behaviors ranged from avoidance to a sincere desire to begin immediately. Both department chairs received phone calls or emails from full- and part-time faculty expressing concern and even fear at the prospect of joining a writing group. They also questioned if they were being forced to join. Many faculty expressed a sincere desire to join such a group, but feared they would have nothing to say or they were not capable of participating in an academic writing group. The majority of concerns raised reflected the tenets of imposter syndrome (Clance & Imes, 1978; Langford & Clance, 1993). Knowledge of the chairs' history of publishing and their willingness to mentor the group calmed many of the anxieties. Once anxieties were allayed, and technical assistance and support were assured, interest increased.

CREATING THE GROUPS

Part of the assessment of interest included asking faculty to list at least three areas in which they would like to publish or conduct research. Once responses were obtained, the chairs reviewed the areas of interest and began the process of pairing faculty with similar interests. BSN and MSN faculty were purposefully comingled in the groups. A balance between faculty who had published and those who had not was also sought to enable senior faculty to guide less experienced faculty through the process of creating their first manuscripts for publication.

A table was created that listed all faculty members and their expressed areas of interest. Once the table was populated, the chairs studied the specific areas of interest and developed large, overarching topics. The purpose was for cross-fertilization of ideas and to ensure that all groups had at least two members, but no more than four or five. Checkmarks were placed under the columns in relation to interested faculty. The writing groups were created by matching faculty with these broader areas of interest.

The chairs served as group facilitators based on their areas of experience. Each chair assigned faculty based on the expressed area of interest as noted in the table. The chairs invited each faculty member to join the group that best represented his or her interest. Approximately 90 percent of the faculty were interested in working in the assigned group. One faculty member asked to be assigned to a different specialty area, stating the redefined group more closely represented her area of interest.

Reasons for declining varied. One faculty member decided that her current work responsibilities did not allow time for participation. Another stated that she was busy writing a dissertation and did not have time. Interestingly, that faculty member joined the first few meetings and the group shared their eagerness to have her participate. They assigned her the responsibility of formatting the first manuscript. She accepted and the group was formed. In the end, she became active in guiding the others and, because of her current research for her dissertation, added greatly to the knowledge base of the group.

ESTABLISHING THE GROUPS AND SELF-SUFFICIENCY

Once the groups were assembled, meetings were set using teleconferencing. During the teleconferences, the chairs explained the writing group process in greater depth. Because each writing group was established with a faculty member who had a track record of publishing, that person was asked to assume the role of facilitator. This approach ensured that each group had immediate access to a member who had experience with the writing and publication process and who was able to guide novice members through the more common pitfalls of writing a first article for publication.

During the initial group meetings, the chairs explained how writing groups worked, offering several suggestions about how a writing group could be established. All of the writing groups decided on assigned roles for each member who would rotate with each new article he or she wrote. The chairs helped to formalize the role of each author. Suggested duties for the role of each author included:

- First author: Establishes contact with the journal, sets deadlines, oversees the group, puts the manuscript in one voice. Often writes the introduction and conclusion and may write the bulk of the article.
- Second author: Conducts and writes the literature review.
- Third author: When research is involved, analyzes the data and writes the results and discussion.
- Fourth author: Ensures that the manuscript is in proper format; contributes as needed.

Each of the three writing groups adopted the suggestions for author roles and, with some modification, applied the suggested duties and roles for their group.

Over time, the writing-group members bonded and supported each other as they planned their manuscripts and refined their topics. As the members of the group became more comfortable, the program chairs slowly stepped back, allowing the writing groups to function independently. Periodically, the writing groups would contact one of the program chairs, requesting advice or to report progress.

RESULTS

The writing groups overcame some major hurdles. These included:

- Time barriers (e.g., living in different time zones across the United States and lack of time to participate)
- Personal and geographic disasters and emergencies (e.g., severe storms causing power loss, preventing members from attending all meetings)
- Diverging ideas on where the writing group should be going (e.g., the majority of members in one group wanted to focus on research while one member wanted to write think pieces; that member decided not to continue with the group)
- Where to submit the manuscript.

At the time of submission of this chapter, one writing group had a manuscript in press. One group decided to conduct research with publication as the penultimate goal. One group has published two articles and two more are in press with a mix of the three authors contributing to the different articles.

CONCLUSION

Creating writing groups with online faculty is one way to assist faculty with professional development, but is a difficult task. Unique barriers present with an online writing group. Not addressing these barriers may lead to frustration and ultimate dissolution of the writing group. Careful mentoring and a solid balance of expert and novice can result in a successful publication.

References

Clance, P. R., & Imes, S. A. (1978). The impostor phenomenon among high achieving women: Dynamics and therapeutic intervention. *Psychotherapy Theory, Research and Practice, 15*, 241–247.

Kittle, P., & Hicks, T. (2009). Transforming the group paper with collaborative online writing. *Pedagogy: Critical Approaches to Teaching Literature, Language, Composition, and Culture, 9*, 525–538.

Langford, J., & Clance, P. R. (1993). The impostor phenomenon: Recent research findings regarding dynamics, personality and family patterns and their implications for treatment. *Psychotherapy, 30*, 495–501. doi: 10.1037/0033-3204.30.3.495

McGrady, L. (2010, May). Hidden disruptions: Technology and technological literacy as influences on professional writing student teams. *The Writing Instructor.* Retrieved from www.writinginstructor.com/mcgrady

Murphy, K. L., Cifuentes, L., & Shih, Y. D. (2004). Online collaborative documents for research and coursework. *TechTrends, 48,* 40–44, 74. doi: 10.1007/BF02763355

Noël, S., & Robert, J.-M. (2003). How the web is used to support collaborative writing. *Behaviour & Information Technology, 22,* 245–262. doi: 10.1080/0144929031000120860

Peterson, C. A., & Umphred, D. A. (2005). A structured faculty development process for scholarship in young faculty: A case report. *Journal of Physical Therapy Education, 19,* 86–88.

Ritchie, S. M., & Rigano, D. L. (2007). Writing together metaphorically and bodily side-by-side: An inquiry into collaborative academic writing. *Reflective Practice, 8,* 123–135. doi: 10.1080/14623940601139087

Staggers, J., Garcia, S., & Nagelhout, E. (2008). Teamwork through team building: Face-to-face to online. *Business Communication Quarterly, 71,* 472–487. doi: 10.1177/1080569908325862